Editor's introduction

Physicians aim to cure diseases or, if that is not possible, to relieve symptoms which interfere with a person's quality of life. Many trials of drug and other therapies use biological end-points (such as a reduction in blood pressure) to determine outcome. There is a growing body of opinion that such outcome measures do not reflect the reality of patient experiences, and measures of 'functional status' or 'health-related quality of life' are appearing with increasing frequency in the medical literature.

It is possible to identify some broad components of health-related quality of life, such as mobility, freedom of pain, mood and so on. Measures such as the Nottingham Health Profile and the Sickness Impact Profile, developed in the UK and USA respectively, have proved successful in tracking the effects of medical and surgical interventions and reflecting apparently more realistically the outcomes of these interventions. However, the multidimensional nature of these scales is perceived by some as a disadvantage, as it is difficult to compare outcomes between patients and across procedures. How can there be a 'trade off', for example, between reduction in pain and depression of mood? There is therefore considerable interest in attempting to value a health state in terms of a single number. Such valuations can then be integrated with the dimension of time in that state to allow comparisons of values achieved by different interventions in different clinical disorders. The best known of these integrated indices is the quality-adjusted life year (QALY), explained in Chapter 3. One immediate implication is that interventions that produce a high number of QALYs per unit cost might be favoured when resources are being allocated.

However, there are a number of scientific and ethical tensions related to measurement of the quality of life. The principal methodological tension is between those who believe that quality of life has so many incommensurable dimensions that it is meaningless to place a single integrated value upon it. Others believe that human beings are perfectly capable of integrating their values and expressing their preferences, as they commonly do in day-to-day life, as judged by their observed behaviour. Then there is discussion as to who should make judgements about the value (utility) of certain dimensions of the life of a person with a particular clinical disorder — the patient who is experiencing the disease, past patients who have experienced both the disease and the treatment, or a sample of the population who have no experience of a disease and who, however well informed, can have little insight into the real nature of the experience of the sufferer. Finally, resources will never be sufficient to provide all the care that might be given, and the allocation of limited resources among different client groups cannot be directed solely upon some mathematical method of measurement, however sophisticated, without the incorporation of both moral and political principles, these last two being occasionally in direct opposition.

The Research Unit of the Royal College of Physicians believes that it may be useful to lay out some of these problems for inspection and further discussion in this book. The potential readership is not only an audience of physicians and economists, but also those interested in the workings of society at large. The chapters in this book were presented for mutual discussion at a Workshop held at the Royal College of Physicians on 10th October 1991.

ANTHONY HOPKINS
Editor

Participants

Indicates authors of papers

***Douglas Black** *Past President, Royal College of Physicians; Convenor, College Committee on Ethical Issues in Medicine, The Old Forge, Duchess Close, Whitchurch on Thames, Reading RG8 7EN.*

Ann Bowling *Needs Assessment Unit, Academic Department of General Practice and Primary Care, The Medical Colleges of St Bartholomew's and the London Hospitals, 2nd Floor, New Science Block, Charterhouse Square, London EC1A 7BE.*

***Martin J. Buxton** *Director, Health Economics Research Group, Brunel, University of West London, Uxbridge, Middlesex UB8 3PH.*

Roy Carr-Hill *School of Social and Political Sciences, University of Hull, Hull HU6 7RX.*

***Michaela J. Cottee** *Quality of Life Research Team, Department of Academic Psychiatry, University College & Middlesex School of Medicine, Riding House Street, London W1N 8AA.*

Jack Dowie *Senior Lecturer, Faculty of Social Sciences, Open University, Walton Hall, Milton Keynes MK7 6AA.*

Lesley Fallowfield *Director, CRC Communication and Counselling Research Centre, London Hospital Medical College, 3rd Floor, Alexandra Wing, Turner Street, London E1 2AD.*

Ray Fitzpatrick *Lecturer in Medical Sociology, Department of Community Medicine and General Practice, Gibson Laboratories, Oxford OX2 6HE.*

Astrid Fletcher *Senior Lecturer in Epidemiology, Division of Geriatric Medicine, Royal Postgraduate Medical School, Hammersmith Hospital, Du Cane Road, London W12 0NN.*

***Howard Glennerster** *Professor of Social Administration, The London School of Economics and Political Science, Houghton Street, London WC2A 2AE.*

***John Grimley Evans** *Professor of Geriatric Medicine, Nuffield Department of Clinical Medicine, Geriatric Medicine Division, Radcliffe Infirmary, Oxford OX2 6HE.*

*Anthony Hopkins *(Organiser and co-Chairman)* *Director, Research Unit, Royal College of Physicians, 11 St Andrews Place, London NW1 4LE.*

*Sonja M. Hunt *Senior Consultant, Galen Research & Consultancy, Southern Hey, 137 Barlow Moor Road, West Didsbury, Manchester M20 8PW.*

*Paul Kind *Centre for Health Economics, University of York, York YO1 5DD.*

Zarrina Kurtz *Consultant in Paediatric Epidemiology, South West Thames Health Authority, 40 Eastbourne Terrace, London W2 3QP.*

Azim Lakhani *Senior Medical Officer, Department of Health, Richmond House, 79 Whitehall, London SW1A 2NS.*

Linda Lamont *Director, The Patients' Association, 18 Victoria Park Square, Bethnal Green, London E2 9PF.*

Michael Lockwood *Department for Continuing Education, University of Oxford, Rewley House, 1 Wellington Square, Oxford OX1 2JA.*

Sally Macintyre *Director, Medical Research Council Medical Sociology Unit, University of Glasgow, 6 Lilybank Gardens, Glasgow G12 8QQ.*

*Stephen McKenna *Senior Consultant, Galen Research & Consultancy, Southern Hey, 137 Barlow Moor Road, West Didsbury, Manchester M20 8PW.*

Henry Neuberger *Department of Health, Room 2812, Millbank Tower, 21–24 Millbank, London SW1P 4QU.*

Christopher Pollitt *Head, Department of Government, Brunel, The University of West London, Uxbridge, Middlesex UB8 3PH.*

*Rosalind Rabin *Quality of Life Research Team, Department of Academic Psychiatry, University College & Middlesex School of Medicine, Riding House Street, London W1N 8AA.*

Nick Ross *34 Kensington Park Road, London W11 3BU.*

*Rachel M. Rosser *Professor of Psychiatry and Head of Department, University College & Middlesex School of Medicine, Wolfson Building, Riding House Street, London W1N 8AA.*

Ian Russell *Director, Health Services Research Unit, University of Aberdeen, Drew Kay Wing, Polwarth Building, Foresterhill, Aberdeen AB9 2ZD.*

*Caroline Selai *Quality of Life Research Team, Department of Academic*

Psychiatry, *University College & Middlesex School of Medicine, Riding House Street, London W1N 8AA.*

***Peter J. Selby** *Director, Institute for Cancer Studies, St James's University Hospital, Leeds LS9 7TF.*

***Clive Smee** *(co-Chairman)* *Chief Economic Adviser, Department of Health, Room 2811, Millbank Tower, 21–24 Millbank, London SW1P 4QU.*

***Paul C. Walker** *Director of Public Health, Norwich District Health Authority, St Andrew's Hospital (North), Yarmouth Road, Norwich NR7 0SS.*

***Alan Williams** *Professor of Economics, Centre for Health Economics, University of York, York YO1 5DD.*

Acknowledgements

The College is grateful to the Department of Health for a contribution to the running costs of the workshop. Administrative assistance and secretarial support to the workshop were provided by Janice Bowman, Barbara Durr and Fiona Shipley. The Research Unit is supported by grants from the Wolfson and Welton Foundations, and other charitable donations.

Contents

1 | How might measures of quality of life be useful to me as a clinician?

Anthony Hopkins
Director, Research Unit, Royal College of Physicians, London

Quality of life and health status

Quality of life embraces many dimensions, ranging from physical well-being and cognitive competence to the establishment of satisfactory interrelationships, the occupation of housing which is enjoyed, and the possession of a sufficient income to explore the world in ways beyond those necessary to ensure basic biological survival.

Figure 1, based upon a figure demonstrated by Eugene Nelson of the New England Medical Center, clarifies the areas of a physician's interest in the quality of life.[1] Factors such as advancing age, income and disappointment in love are all outside a physician's control. Physicians and others in the medical profession are therefore principally concerned with measures of health-related quality of life, or what are usually called measures of health status. A proportion of measured health status reflects the burden of biological disorders, such as

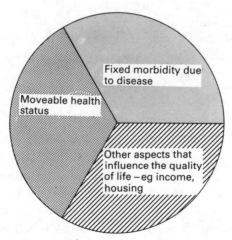

Fig. 1. *Measures of health status.*[1]

Alzheimer's disease and multiple sclerosis, which are probably un-modifiable with present therapies directed at the biological impairment. Another proportion reflects what Nelson has termed 'moveable health status', which is responsive to therapy.

Although I have, as convention indicates, separated out measures of health-related quality of life, it should be noted that a medical intervention can extend into the lower right part of Fig. 1. For example, a neurologist may succeed in persuading a housing authority to rehouse a disabled patient who cannot get down stairs to a ground floor flat from the top floor, thereby considerably reducing his social handicap, and improving the quality of his life.

How might measures of quality of life be useful in routine clinical practice?

The principal task of a clinician is to listen to a patient's symptoms, to identify by physical examination or by investigation any disorder causing the symptoms, to discuss with his patient the available effective treatments and, within the resources available, provide the treatment preferred by his patient. A physician must also determine the outcome that he is trying to achieve. The initially chosen treatment may prove to be only partly effective or ineffective due to some undetermined variable in the patient or his disease, so it may be necessary to modify the chosen therapy.

Measurements of health status are of crucial importance at all stages in this process, yet it is surprising how far medicine has advanced without adequate measurement of functional capacity. On the other hand, measures of biological impairment such as, for example, the fasting blood glucose or measurements of peak expiratory flow are well developed and validated.

I shall use this clinical process of care to illustrate how measures of health-related quality of life (health status) may be useful to a clinician.

Symptoms

First, the clinician listens to a patient's symptoms. When patients describe symptoms such as breathlessness or pain, they do so in the context of their daily social existence: 'I get breathless on going upstairs', or 'I get pain in the upper part of my tummy after eating meals'. They do not come to the physician stating that they have a disease, but rather that the quality of life is impaired in the several ways described. They cannot go upstairs without breathlessness, or they cannot eat meals without discomfort. However, a patient's quality of life may also be impaired by his or her anxiety that he or she might have heart disease or abdominal cancer. Patients want the physician or surgeon to relieve their anxiety, as well as to restore the missing functional ability.

At this stage of a patient career, accurate assessments of functional status are not always necessary or relevant for appropriate clinical action. For example, however mild the abdominal pain, if it be accompanied by a progressive weight loss, a clinician will probably arrange an endoscopic or radiological investigation of the upper gastrointestinal tract: that is to say, a minor degree of impairment of health status may well trigger a major therapeutic action, because of the particular combination of probabilities suggested by points in the history and on examination. An overall measure of functional status therefore is not likely to be useful at this point. Clinicians also routinely make some unmeasured judgements of severity of symptoms and act accordingly. Symptoms perceived by the patient as being severe are more likely to precipitate the arrangement of an investigation or the institution of treatment.

Clinicians may fail to take sufficiently seriously a patient's anxiety about somatic symptoms which do not have a clear basis in structural disease.[2] Measures of impairment of health status that are sensitive to anxiety or emotional well-being therefore have a role to play here. It is hoped that medical schools train physicians to be sensitive to the impairments in social roles caused by illness. A good history will determine how a patient's symptoms are affecting his or her particular domestic life and work. This specific information particular to the patient under discussion is likely to be far more informative than a measure of health status when planning the management of that particular patient's problems.

There are, however, some reasons for introducing a measure of health status into a routine consultation. First, a measure could provide a baseline against which the effectiveness of subsequent interventions could be measured. Secondly, it may well draw attention to some area of impairment that a busy or inexperienced clinician may have overlooked. An example is the presence of depression, a clinical variable known vastly to influence measurements in other domains. Thirdly, it could be argued that a measure of health status applied at the onset of a patient episode could determine the severity of impairment, and therefore the priority that the clinician has to give that particular patient in allocating resources within his or her clinical practice. Clinicians already do this without any particular method of measurement, giving some priority on the waiting list for surgical procedures such as hip replacement to those whom they informally assess as being apparently most disabled. However, for many disorders, the extent of functional impairment is not a matter which determines prioritisation for care, but rather the anxiety about the underlying nature of the biological disease. For example, most surgeons would arrange an early biopsy of a woman's breast lump with skin tethering, even though in itself this will have little effect upon functional status, apart from resulting in understandable anxiety.

Some studies have shown that measures of health-related quality of life correlate poorly with traditional biological measures of impairment. For example, Alonzo has shown that the volume of air that can be expired forcefully in one second (a value known as the FEV_1), a traditional biological measure of airways obstruction, correlates poorly with the patient's self-rated assessment of functional disability.[3] On the other hand, the latter correlates well with his rating of dyspnoea (breathlessness). The traditional approach in biological medicine has been to consider therapies that might reduce the physiological impairment, yet these findings suggest that in this particular example this approach is likely to be of little value, and attention would be better directed towards therapies which improve functional status.

Investigations

The next stage in the career of our patient is often investigation to confirm or refute a hypothetical diagnosis based upon the history and physical examination. Although not strictly a measure of health status, it would seem useful to explore in a more measured way the experiences of what it is like to undergo certain investigations. A recent personal account from a doctor published in the *British Medical Journal* suggests that urologists, for example, underestimate the discomfort caused by a prostatic biopsy.[4] Neurologists seem to underestimate the anxiety caused by prolonged magnetic resonance imaging. There is, I think, a fruitful field of research for the application of some simple measures of patient experiences as new investigative techniques are introduced.

Treatment

The next step in the clinical career outlined above is to discuss with the patient the available treatments for his or her disorder that achieve different outcomes, and to encourage the patient to reach an informed choice, a choice which fully reflects the values that he or she places upon different dimensions of his or her life. For example, even before the relative merits of simple excision of a breast carcinoma were clarified in relation to a radical mastectomy, some women opted for simple excision, valuing their self-image above what was then put to them as a slightly less good chance of survival.

A more recent example is the experience of Wennberg and his colleagues in the USA, who have shown the value of collecting information about outcomes after prostatectomy in routine Medicare practice, and of using those outcomes in discussion with subsequent patients whether to have the operation or wait to see what happens.[5] Wennberg found that 4% of his sample of patients were impotent following surgery. For one patient, the risk of impotence may be of overriding importance in reaching the decision about whether or not to proceed with the operation. For another, because of his life circumstances, the risk may be irrelevant.

This illustrates the need for measures of health status that are focused upon the perspective of the users of health care. Different patients have different values, so it is unlikely that generic measures of health status will necessarily reflect the concerns of individual patients. Furthermore, the focus of patients' interests may alter during the course of their illnesses. Lesley Fallowfield has suggested that a statistically sound method needs to be developed of allowing a patient to determine his or her own quality of life schedule, and to re-rank and re-order items as the disease state changes, and as he or she adjusts to and copes with different problems (personal communication, 1990). This is a goal to which we need to aspire. Meanwhile, a multiplicity of measures that reflect all the domains of health-related quality of life is needed which, by change, can also serve as measures of outcome specific to certain disorders. For example, pain is not a common problem in multiple sclerosis, and would seldom be a suitable measure for this illness. However, people with multiple sclerosis are commonly physically disabled, distressed and incontinent, and any measure of health in this illness should reflect these dimensions.

Research

There are some further areas of medical practice in which measures of health-related quality of life are potentially useful. So far, I have indicated that they can measure the presence and severity of impairment of functional capacity in the psychological and physical domains. A change in health status is a measure of outcome, which may be useful in planning therapy with an individual patient, allowing the patient the expression of patient preferences. A change may also alert a physician to an impairment not suspected from a routine history. In research, measures of health status can be used to monitor the natural history of a disorder, and used as a measure of the impact of therapy.

This includes therapy provided in a routine clinical setting, as well as in randomised controlled trials—in an increasing number of which some measure of health status is used in addition to the more traditional biological variables. For example, a multicentre trial of antihypertensive intervention and management showed that a diet resulting in weight loss benefited the quality of life more than pharmacological therapy, reducing the total number of physical complaints and increasing the subject's satisfaction with health. Furthermore, a weight-reducing diet also ameliorated the adverse effects of pharmacological agents. Blood pressure fell in all trial groups, although atenolol decreased blood pressure substantially more than diet alone.[6] This trial has therefore provided information in an area of health care in which patient choice may in future be pre-eminent. On the face of it, this information suggests that every moderately hypertensive patient should logically choose weight reduction, at least as an ancillary measure to pharmacological therapy. However, many patients might say realistically that previous attempts at weight reduction have failed, that they value their meals with their family and in restaurants over and above the remote risk of a cerebrovascular complication of poorly-treated hypertension, or that they prefer to accept the adverse effects of pharmacological therapy rather than the rigours of weight reduction.

There is, however, a potential tension between using traditional outcome measures and measures of quality of life in randomised controlled clinical trials. For example, many neurologists have always had doubts about the effectiveness of speech therapy following stroke, but most continue to arrange it if possible because, confronted with a severely dysphasic patient, it seems unkind not to do something that might remotely do some good, and certainly could do no harm.[7] However, a controlled trial showed that 'therapy' given by untrained volunteers, usually housewives, under the supervision of a speech therapist was as effective as formal speech therapy, using as an outcome measure a recognised measure of functional communication.[8] On the results of this trial, there is no reason to continue to train speech therapists for work in this field. Another trial would be a comparison of the effectiveness of volunteer 'therapy' against no treatment. A measure of functional communication may show no benefit from the intervention of volunteers (any improvement reflecting merely the natural history of recovery after stroke). However, if a measure of social support and integration were to be used rather than a technical measure of communication, it may well be that the trial would show that the work of volunteers was effective in improving these aspects of life.

As measures of health status become more widely adopted, a decision will need to be made about how many resources can be allocated to supporting our sick population emotionally and in their social integration, even though there is no impact upon the underlying biological disease.

Discharge from hospital

Another area in which measures of health-related quality of life could be useful and helpful to a clinician is in planning a patient's discharge from hospital. A measure of health status that showed considerable physical incapacity would indicate that the patient might not be able to manage in his own home, but would need to be discharged to a nursing home. There is research evidence suggesting that measures of health status do target patients on discharge to a more appropriate system of care than an *ad hoc* assessment based upon clinical impression.[9]

Quality of care

Measures of health status are also of potential use in assuring the quality of care provided by a clinician. Matched for case severity, the achieved outcome health status after an intervention is a measure of the provider's effectiveness of therapy, which potentially may be compared with that of other providers. This approach has been used in intensive care, where one particular measure of health status, the APACHE score, can be used to predict those who have a high probability of surviving their episode of acute illness.[10] If an intensive care unit then has a number of deaths amongst a population of patients who had been predicted to have survived, there should be a review of its processes of care.

Measures of the quality of life can also allow focus of effort where studies using such measures have shown rapid deterioration. For example, in a study of the quality of life of hospice patients before death, measures of the quality of life remained fairly steady until deteriorating sharply in the four weeks preceding death.[11] A sharp deterioration might be used as a predictor of impending death, and changes in the various dimensions of whatever score is used may point up areas in which renewed efforts at effective intervention are required, for example the relief of pain. In this context too, measures of the quality of life may make explicit to both the patient and his or her relatives the trade off between quantity and quality of life. It is well recognised that 'better' terminal care, in the sense of maintaining life of a good quality until the end, may result in a life of a few days shorter duration.

Resource allocation

Clive Smee and others write in later chapters about the use of measures of health-related quality of life in resource allocation, but I would briefly make the following points. Clinicians recognise the right to equal consideration of all sick people, but also recognise that those who are most sick have the greatest needs. Measures of health-related quality of life may prove to be useful in resource allocation in this sense, insofar as a severe impairment of quality of life may justify an early intervention if there is an effective treatment. However, as already mentioned in the case of the hypothetical patient with breast cancer, functional status is not likely to be a pre-eminent variable in clinicians' choice in resource allocation at an individual patient level.

Marketing of services

Finally, as many clinicians have to market their services in the new provider/purchaser culture, measures of health status achieved by interventions may be used in marketing a provider's services.

What do clinicians require of a measure of health status?

To be useful to a clinician, any measurement of health-related quality of life must fulfil the requirements of any other measurement used in clinical medicine. The measure must be *reliable*, consistently measuring what it is meant to be measuring, undeflected to any great extent by chance factors. The test must be *valid*, covering all those dimensions of health-related quality of life that are relevant to the disorder under consideration. We would wish the measure to be *sensitive*, so that patients with significant impairments are identified, and both the effects of progressive illness and the effectiveness of an intervention can be tracked. The measure would also be required to have good *specificity*, discriminating those who are truly experiencing a good health-related quality of life from those who are not. The measure must be *socially acceptable* to patients, *acceptable* to their doctors, and *convenient* to use for those who might be in some way physically impaired, such as partially sighted. An informed clinician would require that the results of such measures were handled in a *statistically appropriate* way — the central tendency of an ordinal scale should not be described by the mean of the ordinal numbers, for example. The measures should be *cheap* to administer and to score, and have *national* and preferably *international* acceptance.

One issue of *Medical Care* was devoted to listing a bibliography of measures of health status, many of which are minor variants upon established ones.[12] These minor variants may well show significant improvements in reliability, validity, specificity and sensitivity over earlier models, but the multiplicity of the scales does to some extent prevent international exchange of information about the effectiveness of treatments. Without in any way setting any choice too rigidly, there would be considerable advantage if the community of health services research workers agreed on a comparatively small number of scales that could form core measures of health status. Whatever other measures were added in any individual research project, these core measures could be included. As an example, the Research Unit of the Royal College of Physicians and the British Geriatrics Society after prolonged discussion have jointly chosen a measure of physical function (the Barthel Score[13]), a measure of cognitive function (the Hodkinson Abbreviated Mental Test[14]), and a measure of mood (the Geriatric Depression Scale[15]), as recommended measures to all those wishing to assess the functional status of the elderly people in their care.[16] With these tools, variations of patterns of care of people with different functional ability may be demonstrated between health districts and, if the measures are sufficiently sensitive, the effectiveness of different types of intervention shown.

What problems do clinicians perceive with the use of measures of quality of life?

The first problem is basically that of unfamiliarity with questionnaires, the design and construction of which do not figure in medical education. Clinicians unfortunately also tend to have a basic distrust of social sciences, regarding data produced by social scientists as 'soft'.[17] Clinicians are unfamiliar with both the high rates of reproducibility of a number of the questionnaires presently available and the considerable variability in laboratory reports, traditionally considered by them to be 'hard' data, such as histopathology and radiology reports. Even when they overcome these prejudices, clinicians are unfamiliar with the significance of the scale scores. Just how 'bad' is a Nottingham Health Profile score of 40, and how much improvement is meant by a subsequent score of 25? There is also the very real problem of the multiplicity of measures of health status from which to choose—and even the market leaders keep changing slightly, thus preventing easy familiarity with one or two 'best buys'.

Another problem is that it is as yet undetermined whether a score of a certain value demands intervention, in the same way that a biopsy report of a possible malignancy demands an intervention. At least one

American hospital has set up a safety net so that patients with very low scores on the psychological health component of a generic measure of health status are reviewed by a psychiatrist.

Then there are technical problems about when to administer a measure of quality of life. To ask a patient to complete a questionnaire one day after he has been told he has cancer is not likely to produce the same results as asking him to complete it two weeks later when he has had a chance to adjust to his new concept of himself and of his illness. Some standardisation of the methodology of administration is definitely necessary.

Many measures of health status reflect functional ability without assistance, which may not reflect the social reality of the situation. For example, to provide a man with a stiff and painful hip with a walking stick may considerably relieve the pain in the hip while he is using the stick, thereby relieving handicap but not disability. As another example, someone who has a caring spouse at home copes very much better with a functional disability than someone who lives alone, so that the quality of life of the former may be very much better even though the scores of physical status are identical.

Measures of health status lack focus, and may obscure factors of prognostic importance to an individual patient. It may well be difficult to link a change in health status to a particular therapeutic intervention. Finally, and most importantly, clinicians are being encouraged to use measures of health status before it has been shown unequivocally that they improve patient care. Few of us doubt the scientific validity of many of the measures of health status, but there is a danger that, like many technologies before them, they may be introduced into routine clinical practice before they have been shown to improve the outcome of medical care.

Clinicians and allocation of resources

In later chapters of this book, there is discussion particularly about who should make the judgements as to resource allocation in terms of improvement of quality of life, but I make some points here from a clinician's perspective.

There is a general perception that doctors have in the past taken too much upon themselves. Most doctors put the perspectives of their own specialties and their own (insufficiency of) information above those of the population of sick people as a whole and of the best research evidence. Who then should allocate resources? It seems improbable that patients suffering with the disorder 'x' can themselves be allowed to determine allocation of resources to treat 'x', as they will be unaware of the conflicting priorities of those suffering with the disorder 'y'. On the other hand, the general population may be insufficiently informed about both disorders 'x' and 'y', or about the reality of living in functional states 'p' and 'q', to determine relative values. It is perhaps for this reason that until recently society trusted a clinician's judgement, as he was presumed to have information about the relative disabilities suffered by clients with functional states 'p', 'q' . . . and disorders 'x', 'y' . . . . Society trusted its physicians to integrate both the likely benefits and the likely adverse outcomes of one or more planned interventions, and then advise the patient clearly as to what, in the light of all matters considered, they judged to be the best course of action. Indeed, the Sidaway case decided that adverse outcomes, however serious, if of only remote probability need not even be mentioned to the patient.[18] Would that judgement be the same today? It may be that such a paternalistic view has gone, possibly for good. The patient and his physician must be in full partnership in deciding upon the right course of action. No one would disagree with this premise, but the reality of the situation is that many patients require help and guidance in reaching a decision about the course to pursue. However carefully the arguments are laid out, some patients may not understand the theory of probability, or the utilities of the various outcomes offered. If I, as a neurologist, had a tight carotid stenosis (more than 70%), I would find it difficult to make an informed decision about whether to have an operation on my neck, with a 10% chance of causing a stroke now, compared to not having an operation and the probability of a 30% chance of a stroke in one year's time.[19] Even retrospective allocation of utility is difficult to think about clearly. A patient who has had an operation which he has survived with a good outcome can safely say he is glad he had that operation, but another patient who had a peri-operative stroke after the same operation can reasonably say that he wishes he had not had it—however, he cannot say what the outcome would then have been because he might have had the stroke anyway.

Conclusion

Griffin has proposed for discussion a concept that well-being is the level to which basic needs are met, but he points out that the definition of 'basic' may vary from person to person.[20] As another proposal, he suggests that 'the level of well-being for any person is in direct proportion to how near that person's life gets to this ideal'. Here then is a pointer to the fact that measures of quality of life cannot by definition be generic, but must be focused upon the individual. People may be disappointed in their chosen careers or in other aspects of their lives about which doctors can do little. Just as the definition of health needs is dependent upon there being an effective treatment for that need—that is, unless there is an effective intervention, there can be no need, only a desire—so it might be said that measures of quality of life are of interest to the health professions only if there is an intervention of proven effectiveness in changing that measure, a measure sensitive to the individual's autonomy and ideals.

Of overriding importance to patients achieving an illness career during which they successfully cope with their symptoms and their meaning is their inner sense of worth, well-being and drive. A neurologist is familiar with patients faced with crippling and progressive neurological disorders who maintain a quiet calm and fortitude in the face of advancing disability. Other patients, with less disability and a far better prognosis are so cast down by what to the external observer appears to be a trivial disorder that they function in life much less well than patients with more severe disorders. Here is a final challenge: how is it possible to measure this drive to competence, a crucial variable in well-being?

References

1.   Nelson E. Presentation at Babson College, Massachusetts, 1990
2.   Creed F, Mayou R, Hopkins A, eds. *Medical symptoms not explained by organic disease*. London: Royal College of Psychiatrists, 1992
3.   Alonzo J. *Measurement of general health status of chronic obstructive pulmonary disease patients*. Presentation at Third Conference on Advances in Health Status Assessment, Washington, 1991
4.   Kelly WP. Better to be forewarned. *British Medical Journal* 1991; **302**: 666
5.   Barry MJ, Mulley AG, Hanley D, Fowler FJ, Wennberg JE, Timothy RP. Symptom status and quality of life following prostatectomy. *Journal of the American Medical Association* 1988; **259**: 3018–22
6.   Wassertheil-Smoller S, Blaufox MD, Oberman A, *et al*. Effect of anti-hypertensives on sexual function and quality of life: the TAIM study. *Annals of Internal Medicine* 1991; **114**: 613–20
7.   Hopkins A. The need for speech therapy following stroke. *Health Trends* 1975; **7**: 58–60
8.   David R, Enderby P, Bainton D. Treatment of acquired aphasia: speech therapists and volunteers compared. *Journal of Neurology, Neurosurgery and Psychiatry* 1982; **11**: 957–61
9.   Williams TF, Hill JG, Fairbank MF, *et al*. Appropriate placement of the chronically ill and aged: a successful approach by evaluation. *Journal of the American Medical Association* 1973; **226**: 1332–5
10. Knaus WA, Draper EA, Wagner DP, Zimmerman JE. An evaluation of outcome from intensive care in major centres. *Annals of Internal Medicine* 1986; **104**: 410–8

11. Morris JN, Suissa S, Sherwood S, Wright SM, Grier D. Last days: a study of the quality of life of terminally ill cancer patients. *Journal of Chronic Diseases* 1986; **39**: 47–62

12. Quality of life: bibliography and indexes. *Medical Care* 1990; **28**: suppl DS 1–DS 77

13. Mahoney FI, Barthel DW. Functional evaluation: the Barthel Index. *Maryland State Medical Journal* 1965; **14**: 61–5

14. Qureschi AN, Hodkinson HM. Evaluation of a ten-question mental test in the institutionalised elderly. *Age and Ageing* 1974; **3**: 152–7

15. Yesavage JA, Brink TL, Rose TL, *et al*. Development and validation of a geriatric depression screening scale—a preliminary report. *Journal of Psychiatric Research* 1983; **17**: 37–49

16. Standardised assessment scales for elderly people. *Report of the Research Unit of the Royal College of Physicians and the British Geriatrics Society*. London: Royal College of Physicians Publications, 1992

17. Deyo R. The quality of life, research and care. *Annals of Internal Medicine* 1991; **114**: 695–6

18. Childs M. Duty to warn of treatment effects. Sidaway vs. the Governors of Bethlem Royal Hospital and others. *Journal of the Medical Defence Union* 1991: **7**: 57–9

19. MRC European carotid surgery trial: interim results for symptomatic patients with severe (70–99%) or with mild (0–29%) carotid stenosis. *Lancet* 1991; **337**: 1235–43

20. Griffin J. *Well-being. Its meaning, measurement and moral importance*. Oxford: Clarendon Press, 1986

2 | How might measures of quality of life be useful to me as a health economist?

Clive Smee
Chief Economic Adviser, Department of Health, London

Quality of life measures in resource allocation

My interest in this field is as Chief Economic Adviser to the Department of Health. The holder of this post is asked to advise on how resources can be allocated as efficiently as possible to serve whatever goals might be set for the health service. Therefore, some key questions to be addressed are whether and how measures of quality of life can be used to improve resource allocation. I see measures of quality of life playing an increasingly important role in the allocation of health resources at several levels.

The national health budget

First, they could strengthen bidding for the overall national health budget. The Treasury's stance in public expenditure negotiations is sensitive to the evidence on the benefits of policy options. At least 40% of total health service expenditure, and probably much more, goes on treatments that have little impact on length of life and must be justified by their contribution to the quality of life in the broadest sense, including the quality of care.

The absence of hard information on the effects of many interventions on quality of life makes them immediately susceptible to Treasury arguments that there is scope for savings. It particularly weakens the arguments for new forms of organising health services, such as community care, as well as undermining arguments for the funding of many new technologies. To provide a better case for the Treasury, it does not matter whether the measures of quality of life are disease-specific or generic. In allocating resources or in negotiating with the Department of Health about the allocation of resources across areas of public expenditure, the Treasury does not see health as a special case. It feels that the same procedures should be used to appraise health expenditures as it tries to apply to roads, railways, education and other areas. Health has to compete, in a sense, within that overall framework.

'The health of the nation'

The second area in which I think better measures of quality of life will be helpful is in setting national priorities under the agenda for *The health of the nation*.[1] This initiative is switching the focus of public policies towards maximising health improvements or health gains and, by implication at least, away from maximising health service activities, particularly acute activities. If the only easily available measures of health and of the impact of various public interventions relate to length of life, there must be a danger that the new targets, both national and local, will be skewed away from areas in which there is need and scope for substantial improvements in the quality of life and care. This point has been made in various ways by people providing evidence during the consultation on *The health of the nation*. Well-respected specific measures of quality of life would help to ensure that areas such as mental health were not left on one side in selecting areas for national targets. Specific measures of quality of life combined with good data on costs would also make it easier to identify the interventions most likely to maximise health gains within particular target areas. Generic measures of quality of life, provided that they enjoy widespread confidence, could help inform choice between target areas.

Purchasers and providers

The third way in which measures of quality of life are becoming increasingly important is through enabling the advantages of separating the roles of purchasers and providers in the health system to be fully exploited. If the new purchasers are to deploy their budget to the greatest health benefit of their member populations, they will require information on the full impacts of different services and interventions. The separation of the purchasing role means that choices based on guesses, prejudices and hope (as they have sometimes been caricatured) are no longer likely to go without challenge. Choices will need to be based, and be seen to be based, on systematic appraisal of the options, as Christopher Pollitt writes in the discussion following Chapter 5. Those decisions or choices that can be backed up by reference to measurable improvements in quality of life will be much easier to defend, though they will doubtless still come under challenge. At this level, both specific and generic measures have an important role to play.

Choices

The fourth area in which I believe measures of quality of life will be important is in informing the choices faced by providers of health services. Some, perhaps many, of these are clinical decisions of the kind discussed in Chapter 1, but there will also be strategic or organisational decisions that could benefit from more information on the impact of alternative options on patient quality of life.

Quality of life measures in decision making

I have referred several times to the 'role' that measures of quality of life could play in decision making at various levels. It may be worth spelling out a little what that role might be, and—more importantly perhaps—what I believe it is not likely to be.

Across the public sector there is general acceptance, at least in government, that policy options should be considered within a broad cost-benefit framework (I emphasise the word 'broad'). In some areas, for example transport, this framework is more rigorously developed and quantified than in others, such as health. This approach emphasises the importance of quantifying impacts, outcomes or effects wherever possible, and of describing qualitatively those impacts for which it has not yet been possible to derive quantitative measures or values. Measures of quality of life could be seen as one way of extending the range of effects or impacts from health interventions for which it is possible to derive quantitative measures. If the impacts on different aspects of both the quality of life and the length of life can be brought together in a single, weighted measure, judgements are further simplified. But—and it is a big 'but'—as in other policy areas, the speed of movement in this direction will depend on there being a consensus on the appropriate sets of weights.

Conclusion

It seems unlikely that measures of quality of life, however comprehensive, will ever be more than one factor to be taken into account when comparing policy options. There will always be other concerns, as some of the following chapters point out, such as equity, access, and burdens on carers. The role of generic measures such as quality-adjusted life years (QALYs) is likely to be further restricted, in my view, by their necessarily partial coverage of the different dimensions of the quality of life. The current crudity of such measures, and the inevitably contentious nature of the weightings, suggest that at present they may be best seen as sources of challenge to incrementalist approaches to the distribution of health service resources. They can certainly facilitate a lively debate over priorities, including waiting list priorities, between purchasers and providers, economists and clinicians, and economists and economists—in fact, between most groups of the population. While their role may become more important, I believe that measures of quality of life are never likely to determine resource allocations: they will always be decision aiding, not decision making.

Reference

1.   Department of Health. *The health of the nation*. London: HMSO, 1991

DISCUSSION

Nick Ross: As someone from outside both medicine and economics, may I ask whether there is an overwhelming consensus within medicine that resources are limited and therefore prioritisation is essential? No unit or regional managers have been invited to contribute to this publication, which seems to me perhaps an omission. These are the people who above all are having to make decisions about resource allocation—by above all, I mean above clinicians at the moment.

I know of a case where the medical profession is combining to try to prevent the closure of a hospital which, looking at the decision as a journalist, seems an eminently sensible management decision. A better quality of clinical care could be provided for less expense if the hospital were to be closed and the patients moved to a larger hospital with better facilities and better resources. I do not detect that there is within the clinical environment an overall acceptance of the need to prioritise resources sensibly. Without consensus, the debate about QALYs and so forth becomes rather academic. Should we not simply tell the doctors to get on with it, give all their resources to the first patient who comes in the door, or in whatever way they want to distribute them? How far is this culture of spreading resources carefully and thoughtfully diffused throughout the medical community?

Paul Walker: Directors of Public Health are probably the main technical advisers when a health authority sets priorities. I regard myself as a manager, though I am not called one. Nine per cent of the gross national product seems to meet some sort of balance between supply and demand, so it could be argued that 33% or perhaps 50% more resources are needed. However, doctors have been used to restrained resources since 1948 and before, and are well aware of priorities. Clinicians tackle resource allocation by a political process, often behind closed doors, not in a transparent way. I think we should try to make the whole process more transparent.

Ian Russell: I judge that there is an increasing acceptance of the need to order priorities in Scotland. A snapshot view now may suggest that many clinicians do not yet accept this need, but an increasing number of them do.

Zarrina Kurtz: From experience in my regional health authority, I think that there is still a substantial difference in understanding between clinicians and public health physicians, or between those who are used to looking at the needs of their patients from a population perspective and those who treat the individual. This gives rise to conflict, even among clinicians within the same specialty, as the pace of change differs. For example, community paediatricians are more aware of the population perspective than acute paediatricians in the experience of those responsible for purchasing child health services.

In our region we work explicitly with agencies other than the National Health Service, principally the social services, because we understand that if health gain is to be demonstrated in terms of quality of life for our population, other agencies have an important input. Many physicians realise that gains in quality of life can often come only from agencies over which they have no control, and with which they have so far not necessarily worked very well. Our colleagues in social services, housing and transport will all contribute to gains in health-related quality of life.

Peter Selby: There is really not so much a difference in pace between community physicians and practising acute physicians, but more a gulf in understanding. I speak from two standpoints. First, wearing my quality of life measurement and planning hat as a physician helping prepare our regional strategic response to *The health of the nation* initiative, I am used, within that forum, to listening to a broad acceptance that we are working in a period of overt as opposed to previously covert rationing. Secondly, in the clinical community, within which I work as an active cancer physician, there is no acceptance that overt rationing is something that should be accepted widely. Clinicians are not particularly tense and angry about this, but there is an anxiety within the clinical community that the gulf between clinicians and those who allocate resources is not necessarily a gulf of ignorance on their part alone. They perceive that precise answers are being sought by health administrators to guide major decisions in allocating resources, and have serious concerns—as I do—that the information is not being sought in a precise, effective, scientific or particularly valuable way.

3 | The present state of play about QALYs

Alan Williams and Paul Kind
Centre for Health Economics, University of York

Introduction

No country can now afford to undertake all the health care activities that might be of some benefit to someone at some time. Priorities therefore have to be established between the activities that should be undertaken and those which should not, at least for the time being. If the resources available for health are to be used in such a way as to maximise the health of the community served, a *generic* measure of health is needed which enables a wide range of health care activities to be compared in a systematic way. To be of practical use, such a measure must be reducible to a single index, even though it may—indeed should—be made up of components which reflect the multi-dimensional nature of health. In other words, a generic summary measure of the benefits of health care activities in terms of individual health outcomes is needed, which also represents the relative value attached by society to different improvements in health. Other things being equal, resources should flow into activities yielding large benefits per unit of resource used, at the expense of those yielding small benefits per unit of resource used.

The quality-adjusted life year (QALY) claims to be such a generic measure of health benefit. This chapter will concentrate on research activity in the UK explicitly concerned with the development of quality-of-life measurement for use in the calculation of QALYs, and will consider:
— the essential characteristics of the quality-adjusted life year;
— the description of health-related quality of life;
— the valuation of health states;
— reaching a group valuation;
— ethics and equity;
— conclusions.

Coverage of these topics has to be selective because of space constraints.

The essential characteristics of the quality-adjusted life year

A careful distinction needs to be made between the process of measuring quality of life and the specific application of such measurement in the computation of QALYs. The integration of data on the quality of life with corresponding data on life expectancy yields a single index of health benefit, expressed in terms of QALYs. It is this combination of data on quality and quantity of life in a single index value which distinguishes QALYs from other forms of measure of benefit. Our interest in life expectancy *and* in quality of life arises from the notion that health care can influence either or both of these. Clinicians and patients often have to trade one against the other. The research problem is how best to represent this process, and to make explicit the implied valuations of all parties concerned. The primary intention is to provide policy makers with information that can be used in setting priorities at both clinical and managerial levels in the National Health Service (NHS).

In order to elicit this trade off, it is necessary for the states of being healthy and of being dead to enter into the process of valuation. There is no requirement that the latter be the worst conceivable state, or that quality of life be described or the valuations elicited in any particular way or from any particular sort of person, or that they be brought together in any particular way. The only *sine qua non* is that being healthy and being dead be amongst the states that are valued relatively to each other, for only then can length of life be systematically valued relatively to quality of life in the QALY framework. It is important to stress this at the outset, because many commentators seem to confuse the *concept* of the QALY with its empirical manifestations thus far,[1,2] which in the UK have been largely based on Rosser's pioneering work from the early 1970s,[3,4] which was not intended at the time for use in QALY calculations.[5]

Any researcher entering this field has several important strategic choices to make:
— how is health-related quality of life to be *described*?
— how are different health states to be *valued* relatively to each other?
— how are individuals' values to be transformed into a *group* value?

There is no reason why every researcher should make the same choice. Eventually, therefore, there may well be as many different approaches to measuring QALYs as there are currently to measuring quality of life, and the choice will rest on their appropriateness for the purpose in hand. We will explain the choices we have made, but others have made different choices (eg Torrance and Feeny in Canada,[6] and Bergner[7] and Kaplan[8] in the USA). It is open to those who think some other route more promising or appropriate to test it out, but if they are to address the issue of setting priorities for the NHS in outcome terms they will have to work within the QALY concept, however broad it may be.

There is, in fact, a fourth strategic decision to be made, namely, *whose* values are to be elicited and used. This decision is not for the researcher to make, but the policy maker. Among the possible candidates are the values of current or recent patients, relatives, doctors, nurses, managers, health authority members, and the general public. Researchers need to explore how far any differences in the relative valuations assigned to health states are explicable with respect to personal background characteristics such as the different roles people may play, plus age, sex, marital status, income, education, religious beliefs, social class and other variables. None was found in our pilot data.

The description of health-related quality of life

If health is assumed to be a concept that has more than one dimension, the *description* of health-related quality of life requires, first, a choice of dimensions or domains and, secondly, a decision about the number of categories or levels of goodness/badness within each dimension or domain. *These choices have to be made with all measures of quality of life.* The particular features relevant to QALYs which are intended to assist priority setting in the NHS are that the descriptors must not be either condition- or treatment-specific. Furthermore, if the valuations of the general public are to be elicited, these descriptors need to be cast in terms that ordinary people can understand and to which they can respond. The theoretical universe of possible health states must not be so large that deriving a set of valuations would be impracticable. The option of restriction to a profile of health states would not allow the priority-setting problem outlined in the introduction to be set.

As mentioned earlier, our work hitherto has been based on Rosser's classification of illness states (see Table 1). This contains seven categories of disability and four of distress which, together with the states of being unconscious and dead, generate a total of 30 possible health states. Rosser's elaboration of this classification is outlined in Chapter 7. Other people in the UK working towards a single index have adopted a different approach. Buxton and colleagues at Brunel have used 'scenarios' which include brief details of past symptoms and treat-

Table 1. Rosser's classification of illness states.[3]

Disability	Distress
1. No disability	**A.** No distress
2. Slight social disability	**B.** Mild
3. Severe social disability and/or slight impairment of performance at work	**C.** Moderate
Able to do all housework except very heavy tasks	**D.** Severe
4. Choice of work or performance at work very severely limited	
Housewives and old people able to do light housework only but able to go out shopping	
5. Unable to undertake any paid employment	
Unable to continue any education	
Old people confined to home except for escorted outings and short walks and unable to do shopping	
Housewives able only to perform a few simple tasks	
6. Confined to chair or able to move around in the house only with support from an assistant	
7. Confined to bed	
8. Unconscious	

ments. This is obviously unsuitable for our particular purposes, since the results become condition- and treatment-specific. Buckingham at Aberdeen is currently using the short-form 36 questionnaire developed for the Medical Outcomes Study, supplemented by vignettes.[9]

In addition to this work centred in the UK, the Middlesex, Brunel and York groups are collaborating in a European enterprise which has been developing a descriptive system designed to abstract key salient features of health-related quality of life for use alongside whatever other measures of outcome might be employed in a particular study.[10] By using the same system for describing this common core of quality of life

Table 2. The Euroqol© descriptive system (as at the date of the three surveys).[10]

Mobility
1. No problems walking about
2. Unable to walk about without a stick, crutch or walking frame
3. Confined to bed

Self care
1. No problems with self care
2. Unable to dress self
3. Unable to feed self

Main activity
1. Able to perform main activity (eg work, study, housework)
2. Unable to perform main activity

Social relationships
1. Able to pursue family and leisure activities
2. Unable to pursue family and leisure activities

Pain
1. No pain or discomfort
2. Moderate pain or discomfort
3. Extreme pain or discomfort

Mood
1. Not anxious or depressed
2. Anxious or depressed

For convenience, each composite health state has a six-digit code number relating to the relevant level of each dimension, with the dimensions always listed in the order given above. Thus, 112232 means:
1. No problems walking about
1. No problems with self care
2. Unable to perform main activity
2. Unable to pursue family and leisure activities
3. Extreme pain or discomfort
2. Anxious or depressed

information across a wide range of studies, it is hoped to render comparable the otherwise non-comparable results of studies conducted in different countries using different measures of quality of life. This Euroqol© descriptive system is still being developed. One version is shown in Table 2. It has recently been decided to adopt the Euroqol© descriptive system in future work at York.

The valuation of health states

The *valuation* of health states is required to generate quality adjustments on a scale in which dead = 0 and healthy = 1. Negative values are possible if any states are regarded as worse than being dead. Various techniques are available for generating such valuations, all of which have weaknesses, and there is no 'gold standard'. Each tends to give somewhat different results, and they vary in their demands upon both respondents and those administering the questionnaires. They can be costly to administer because of the complexity of the protocols required to meet these demands. The methods include:

1. *Magnitude estimation*, in which people are asked to say how many times worse is state A than state B.
2. *Category rating*, which comes in many variants. The one used mainly by ourselves and the Euroqol© group is a visual analogue scale in the form of a thermometer (Fig. 1). People are asked to indicate on the thermometer how good or bad are various states.
3. *Time trade off*, in which people are asked how many years in a state of good health they regard as equivalent to a stated number of years in some specified state of poor health. The bigger the sacrifice of life expectancy they are willing to make, the worse the poor health state is assumed to be valued.
4. *Standard gamble*, in which people are asked what risk of immediate death they would be willing to accept to escape from a specified poor state of health and to achieve good health — the bigger the acceptable risk, the worse the poor health state must be valued.

In her original work, Rosser used the magnitude estimation method, but in more recent work she has been using the standard gamble. The Brunel group used time trade off, and Buckingham, at Aberdeen, is currently experimenting with an innovatory version of this technique in which the trade off is of time *within a day*. The Euroqol© group adopted the thermometer version of category rating, because it seems the most practicable in postal questionnaires. At York we are still relatively uncommitted, but have dropped magnitude estimation. In the next phase of the work we shall concentrate on establishing the relative

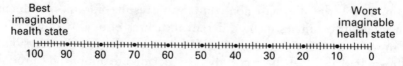

Fig. 1. *The Euroqol© thermometer.*[10]

merits (at an empirical level) of the time trade off and standard gamble methods, using the following criteria:

— *face validity*: the intuitive appeal of the nature of the choice confronting participants;
— *comprehensibility*: the extent of participants' understanding of the valuations task;
— *internal consistency*: the extent to which the valuations conform to the logically indicated order;
— *reliability*: the extent to which participants' initial responses are replicated when asked to repeat each valuation task;
— *experimental burden*: the ease with which subjects and interviewers complete the task, and the time taken to collect the data.

The pilot valuations derived by the Euroqol© group (Table 3) show remarkable similarity between respondents in England, the Netherlands and Sweden, though it remains to be seen whether these preliminary results will be sustained in bigger surveys, and whether they are found also, say, in the Mediterranean countries. Rosser's original valuations (Table 4) are well-known. We have recently revalued the states in her original classification system using nearly 300 members of

Table 3. Median valuations from three surveys.[10]

| Health state | Median valuations | | |
	Lund (Sweden)	Frome (England)	BoZ (Netherlands)
111111	100	99	95
111121	86	84	86
111112	75	70	75
111122	70	68	70
112121	65	70	65
112131	50	59	60
112222 (a)	35	40	43
112222 (b)	39	40	40
112232	35	35	33
212232	22	25	20
222232	10	10	7
232232	7	5	6
322232	4	2	5
332232	1	1	4
being dead (a)	0	0	3
being dead (b)	0	1	2

Two valuations are reported (a and b) for the states that were repeated on successive pages of the questionnaire.

Table 4. Rosser's original matrix (all 70 subjects).[3]

Disability rating	Distress rating			
	A (None)	**B** (Mild)	**C** (Moderate)	**D** (Severe)
1. None	1.000	0.995	0.990	0.967
2. Slight social	0.990	0.986	0.973	0.932
3. Severe social or slight work	0.980	0.972	0.956	0.912
4. Work severely limited	0.964	0.956	0.942	0.870
5. Unable to work	0.946	0.935	0.900	0.700
6. Confined to chair	0.875	0.845	0.680	0.000
7. Confined to bed	0.677	0.564	0.000	−1.486
8. Unconscious	−1.028	Not applicable		

the general public as respondents in place of her 70 (a mixture of doctors, nurses, patients and healthy volunteers). The time trade off and thermometer methods have been used, as well as the magnitude estimation method, to elicit valuations.

Because of various weaknesses in the design of our pilot study, the results are difficult to interpret, but they are very different from Rosser's (Table 5). The values for each state according to each method are shown in Table 5, some of which manifest 'reversals' in the sense that the expected rank order of valuations has been violated. Where a state is involved in such a reversal, the valuation is enclosed in brackets. Reversals seem to be due to a variety of factors, prominent amongst which is the fact that for logistic reasons each individual valued only a subset of the states. Thus, when put together in a single matrix they represent the valuations of different subsets of people. Moreover, some individuals appear to regard 'moderate' as better than 'mild'. Others seem to have had considerable difficulties in coping with the valuation task, but their data were left in rather than rejected as 'unusable', as seems to have been the practice of some earlier researchers in this field.* To make it easier for those disinclined to disentangle such

*The data are all available to researchers via the Survey Research Archive of the Economic and Social Research Council.

Table 5. Synthesised valuation matrix. Synthesised values (derived by personal judgement) from the medians of individually transformed data elicited by ME, TTO and CR valuation methods.

Disability states	Distress states			
	A	**B**	**C**	**D**
1	[1.00]	.89 .90 .85 --------------- .90	.89 .80 .85 --------------- .85	.67 .45(.35) --------------- .55
2	.89 .90 .85 --------------- .90	.81 .70(.45) --------------- .70	.78(.60)(.60) --------------- .60	.56 .35(.50) --------------- .45
3	.70(.55)(.50) --------------- .65	.63 .53 .44 --------------- .55	.57(.55)(.30) --------------- .50	.44 .20 .30 --------------- .35
4	.63(.70)(.55) --------------- .60	.56(.45).42 --------------- .50	.51(.55)(.40) --------------- .45	.40 .33 .22 --------------- .30
5	.44 .55(.25) --------------- .50	(.43).45(.35) --------------- .40	(.44)(.43)(.26) --------------- .35	.22 .20 .17 --------------- .20
6	.44 .43(.41) --------------- .40	(.44)(.45)(.39) --------------- .35	.34(.45)(.30) --------------- .30	.22 .15 .14 --------------- .15
7	(.38).20 .20 --------------- .30	(.40).10(.16) --------------- .25	.33 .03(.20) --------------- .20	.20[neg].0 --------------- .10
8	.01	[neg]		.00
		00		

The data in each cell are as follows:

ME	TTO	CR
Synthesised		

Parentheses indicate that the state was one of a pair manifesting inconsistency. ME = magnitude estimation; TTO = time trade off; CR = category rating.

complex data, but who are committed to Rosser's original descriptive
system and seek valuations likely to be closer to those of the general
public, a common sense synthesis has been suggested for use in place of
her original matrix.

Reaching a group valuation

The data presented above are the product of an important step which
deserves closer attention in all measures of quality of life (and indeed in
all outcome measures), which invariably involve grouping individual
data into some overall measure. Transforming individual values into a
group value is often mistakenly seen as a purely technical matter, the
choice of measure of central tendency supposedly depending wholly on
the characteristics and shape of distribution of the data—but it is
actually an important political act, for it determines the weight to be
given to each person's views.

Although the choice of measure of central tendency is a pervasive
problem throughout measurement of the quality of life, it seems to
surface only in discussions of QALYs. On technical grounds, the
median value has often been chosen as the appropriate measure of
central tendency, since the data may not be normally distributed. This
is also politically appropriate in a system in which decisions are made
by simple majority vote, for then the median voter is decisive. Value
judgements are made even in such an apparently straightforward
criterion for choosing between treatments based on the two-year
survival rate. This 'average' concept carries the implicit assumption
that every survivor counts equally, that to survive less than two years is
(on average) of no value to anyone and, having survived two years,
further survival is (on average) also of no further value to anyone.
These are all strong assumptions.

Some people may be tempted to take an even more extreme position:
since people's values are diverse, no measure of central tendency
should be used, but everyone should be treated in accordance with their
own values. This would be defensible only if the decisions being made
had no implications for anyone other than the person whose values
were being considered. In a world of scarcity and opportunity cost,
however, this is never true: choosing to treat one person necessarily
implies not treating some other person(s). The values of every affected
or potentially affected person are surely relevant. Since it will not
normally be known who the untreated persons are, there is little option
but to use some 'representative' set of values. Moreover, in a tax-
financed system of health care the views of those providing resources

through taxes, who are also potential patients in the long run, may also carry some weight. Thus, at the level of policy, clinical as well as managerial, a group value will be required based on some measure of central tendency. It will not necessarily be the same group whose values are held to be relevant to every decision, nor will the same measure of central tendency always be appropriate, but the use of some such measure cannot be avoided. Group decisions require group values.

Ethics and equity

Most QALY calculations are based on the assumption that a QALY is of equal value no matter who is the beneficiary, but there is nothing inherent in the QALY concept that requires this simple assumption. If it were felt more appropriate to weight benefits to the young more heavily than those to the elderly, or to the parents of young children more heavily than to childless people,[11] there is no reason in principle why such weights should not be incorporated into the calculations, although there may well be some formidable empirical problems in eliciting such weights.[12] Thus, much of the criticism of the allegedly inherent inequity of QALYs is mistaken, but there are some wider ethical issues that deserve more careful consideration.

QALYs are based on the fundamental assumptions, first, that the objective of the NHS is to improve people's health and, secondly, that the relevant notion of health to use in this context is life expectancy and quality of life, as valued in some socially approved manner, for example, by the median view of the general public, using such equity weights as are considered appropriate. QALYs are therefore of relevance to the extent that the NHS adopts this essentially consequentialist position. However, this seems equally true of *all* quality of life measures, as well as survival rates and all other outcome measures, so it is not peculiar to QALYs.

Other fundamental assumptions are possible, and the more important they are held to be, the less weight will be given to QALYs and all other outcome measures. The most common of these other assumptions are those that focus on process rather than outcome, arguing, for example, that people are entitled to some minimum level of care even if it does them little, or even no, good in terms of improving the length or quality of their life.[13] Another common argument is that people who are otherwise deprived should get privileged access to health care to compensate them for the bad deal fate has handed out to them.[14] If these alternative positions are indeed accepted by the general public as important additional objectives of the NHS, it should be recognised that their acceptance implies that the overall health of the population will be worse than it need have been. People *on average* will both die sooner and suffer more than they need have done.

For completeness, one further line of argument that must be mentioned is the assertion that *any* discrimination that involves one person sitting in judgement upon the worth of someone else's life and, by implication, upon the value of changes in the length or quality of someone else's life, is morally repugnant and must be avoided. Since it is acknowledged that choices have to be made, it is argued that the only ethical way to make them is by lottery. Unfortunately, such arguments usually stop there, with no guidance offered as to how this lottery is to be designed in such a way that the people responsible for its design can avoid making the same discriminatory judgements that the lottery was supposed to avoid.[15] It is also curious that these arguments are typically levelled against QALYs, but not against survival rates or scores on measures of quality of life, despite these too being used to choose between treatments and between who shall and shall not be treated. Other measures too involve implicit judgements about the relative worth of different people's lives. The reality of clinical practice is that such judgements are made daily.

Conclusions

As pointed out at the outset, the distinctive feature of QALYs is the trade off between length and quality of life because all the other aspects also occur elsewhere in measurement of the quality of life. There is no doubt that this particular trade off is extremely difficult to elicit in a reliable and systematic manner. Indeed, it seems to be the major research problem in the QALY field, but the alternative to attempting to find out the sort of trade off individuals appear willing to make is to measure life expectancy and quality of life separately, and leave it to the policy makers (clinical or managerial) to establish the trade off, implicitly or explicitly, on behalf of the individuals concerned. This happens every time a doctor asserts that some risk associated with treatment is 'acceptable', or is so small as not to be worth mentioning. The time trade off and standard gamble methods both attack the life-expectancy versus quality-of-life problem fairly directly, and seem the best of the available ways forward in this difficult territory.

There is a great deal still not known about the measurement and valuation of health-related quality of life. The QALY, being the most ambitious of the concepts attempting to determine quality of life, exposes (and is vulnerable to) most such gaps in our knowledge. At the fairly primitive stage at which we currently find ourselves, two important strategic questions are raised:

1. Does the present generation of QALY measures represent a sufficient improvement over existing methods of priority setting in health care to find a place in the armamentarium and, if so, what is that place? This question is addressed in Chapter 4 by Martin Buxton, and by others in discussion.
2. In what order of priority should the deficiencies in our present knowledge be tackled? Unfortunately, this question is not addressed in this book, perhaps because it is too large and too technical, but it needs to be addressed seriously and realistically in relation to the research capacity available.

References

1. Williams, A. The economics of coronary artery bypass grafting. *British Medical Journal* 1985; **291**: 325–9
2. Gudex C. Prioritising waiting lists. *Health Trends* 1990; **3**: 103–8
3. Rosser RM, Watts VC. The measurement of hospital output. *International Journal of Epidemiology* 1972; **1**: 361–8
4. Rosser RM, Kind P. A scale of valuations of states of illness—is there a social consensus? *International Journal of Epidemiology* 1978; **7**: 347–58
5. Rosser RM. From health indicators to quality adjusted life years: technical and ethical issues. In: Hopkins A, Costain D, eds. *Measuring the outcomes of medical care*. London: Royal College of Physicians of London & King's Fund Centre for Health Services Development, 1990: 1–17
6. Torrance GW, Feeny D. Utilities and quality adjusted life years. *International Journal of Technology Assessment in Health Care* 1989; **5**: 559–75
7. Bergner M. Development, testing and use of the sickness impact profile. In: Walker SR, Rosser RM, eds. *Quality of life: assessment and application*. Lancaster: MTP Press, 1988
8. Kaplan RM, Anderson JP. The quality of well-being scale: rationale for a single quality of life index. In: Walker SR, Rosser RM, eds. *Quality of life: assessment and application*. Lancaster: MTP Press, 1988
9. Buckingham Quality Quest Inc. SF36 system, 1989
10. Euroqol© Group. Euroqol©—a new facility for the measurement of health-related quality of life. *Health Policy* 1990; **16**: 199–208.
11. Charny MC, Lewis PA, Farrow SC. Choosing who shall not be treated in the NHS. *Social Science and Medicine* 1989; **28**: 1331–8
12. Williams A. Ethics and efficiency in the provision of health care. In: Bell JM, Mendus S, eds. *Philosophy and medical welfare*. Cambridge: Cambridge University Press, 1988: 111–26
13. Carr-Hill RA. Allocating resources to health care: is the QALY (quality adjusted life year) a technical solution to a political problem? *International Journal of Health Services* 1991; **21**: 351–72

14. Harris J. QALYfying the value of life. *Journal of Medical Ethics* 1987; **13**: 117–23
15. Williams A. QALYs or short straws. *British Medical Journal* 1986; **293**: 337–8

DISCUSSION

Sally Macintyre: More information than has been supplied so far is needed, not about the arguments why QALYs should be used, but about who, if anybody, is using them, for what purposes, and with what consequences. Clive Smee discussed the role they *might* play and how they *might* be used, and Alan Williams has talked about how they *should* be used — but I am not yet clear whether anybody is actually using them. This is something that I would like to have discussed. Alan Williams distinguishes the concepts of QALYs with their empirical uses to date. He is perhaps suggesting that much of the criticism of those concepts is based on imperfections of the method so far, but I am not sure whether the principle can be separated from the practice in this way, and whether we can say they are good in theory and that the practicalities of using them have to be ignored. While it might be desirable to have generic measures with all the attributes that Alan Williams suggests, they are of no use if they prove empirically, conceptually, politically and ethically difficult — and, in fact, impossible — to use, or if people do not agree about them when they try to use them.

In informing us about the present situation with QALYs, Alan Williams has given an eloquent description of them and what he hopes to achieve from their use. My view about the current position is that, compared with the rigorous and extensive developmental work that has gone into many other quality of life measurements, there is a surprisingly small empirical and conceptual basis for the QALY methodology. Many policy makers would probably be surprised both to discover the poor empirical underpinning of the measures, and to hear that the original valuations are those of a selected group of only 70 people.

In the material on Euroqol© described by Alan Williams at the workshop, I was surprised and slightly appalled by the very low response rates to the questionnaires asking people to value different states of health. Many of the questionnaires that were returned had to be discarded, which suggests that people either did not understand them or had other problems with them.

Therefore, at the moment, my view of the current state of play about QALYs is that we are still at the stage of arguing about whether they are a good tool in theory. More needs to be known about whether they are good in practice, but I do not know whether this can be divorced from questions about the empirical and conceptual underpinning of the measures presently used. Enthusiasm for using QALYs has, I feel, rather outstripped their practical development and application.

Astrid Fletcher: So far, the problems of construction of health indices, valuation and low response rates have been emphasised. There has been little discussion about the desirability, or indeed the appropriateness, of combining quality of life with life expectancy. When quality and quantity of life are aggregated, the assumption is made that these are equivalent, that years of life gained are valued equally with the quality of life of those years. This may or may not be much of a problem philosophically, but it is a problem when life expectancy and quality are aggregated over individuals. The scenario then suggested by one QALY represents by this integration a large number of options which are not made either explicit or clear. QALYs are not understood by many people, including clinicians, physicians, and buyers of health care, who may not understand how survival is integrated with quality of life. The integration causes confusion between the large range of available options when people are making decisions about the resources they should buy. Thus, a purchaser of health care might opt for treatments which give the best costs per QALY, but which have very different implications in terms of the relative weightings of survival and quality of life. For example, Martin Buxton points out in Chapter 4 that a gain of 20 QALYs to one individual is, by definition, of equal value to a gain of one QALY to 20 individuals, but the differences are more than that—they represent different scenarios. For example, the highest number of QALYs may be derived from a treatment associated with a very poor survival in some patients, but with a very good quality of life in the survivors compared to another treatment with less benefit for quality of life but fewer adverse effects on survival. There is a huge range of options in one QALY, which cannot be made explicit unless the dimensions of survival, life expectancy and quality of life are teased out and presented separately. I believe that it is extremely misleading to present a QALY as a single summary statistic.

Furthermore, to take one example with which I am familiar, all apparent benefits of treating mild hypertension in terms of life years gained can be removed by changing the utility value for adverse effects of treatment from 0.99 to 0.98. This illustrates the dramatic effects of small changes in valuations of health states. In my view, these calculations say nothing about the overall effects of side-effects against the benefits of antihypertensive treatment, but only that a methodology is being used which has not yet been properly worked out.

Alan Williams: I think it is best to keep separate the issues of the integration of life expectancy and quality of life for an individual and how the measures for different individuals are added together.

I think we have to press on with the integration of life expectancy and quality of life at the level of an individual because individuals face these choices, for example, every time they undergo surgery. They are accepting risks of peri-operative mortality against promised improvements in quality of life. People are continually facing those risks, so it is important to find out about the trade offs established between them.

With regard to adding such measures together, Astrid Fletcher said that an individual can score, say, three QALYs, which can be achieved in a number of different ways — which means that the task I set out to address has in fact been addressed correctly. The purpose was to find a common rubric within which the benefits of different things can be compared. At some level in the decision-making process, we may indeed want to disaggregate this, and say that those three QALYs derived from an improvement in quality of life, in the sense of increased mobility and reduced pain for an old lady with osteoarthritis of the hip, whilst they were gained by increasing the life expectancy of somebody with breast cancer by five years — and so on. At one level, we want to know how each QALY was achieved, and that additional information should always be recoverable from the original data.

The question to be addressed is how much information can be processed by people at different levels in the hierarchy of health care. It is not surprising that a change in valuation of health states in treated hypertension brought about a dramatic change in the preferred treatment for hypertension. If the changes in the valuations do not change anything, why have them? There has to be some critical point at which a change in the valuations used changes the preferred outcome.

Anthony Hopkins: The illustration Astrid Fletcher used in relation to hypertension is crucial to our understanding because, if variations in the valuations of health states have such an enormous and apparently unrealistic impact upon the QALY calculations, this comes back to the methodological issues that are part of the subject under discussion. Valuations of health states may not yet be sufficiently robust to be used in the field.

Paul Kind: In response to Astrid Fletcher, what is so fundamental about the notion of reducing information to a single index and aggregating across different domains? I find it difficult to understand the basis on which that objection is lodged. In subsequent discussions, we might further elaborate the extent to which there is an objection to the notion of the conceptual basis of this work, that the so-called health-related quality of life measures are themselves conceptually without basis and not measuring something significant and useful.

Lesley Fallowfield: I am concerned about the way in which people at meetings about budget allocations are seduced by slick graphs and tables. People tend to believe them, rather than question (as Sally Macintyre pointed out) the data used to produce those calculations. I, too, am worried, particularly about the instruments currently being used at York. They have had little testing of validity and reliability, as would be demanded of any of the quality of life tools presently used in clinical trials.

Clive Smee: Sally Macintyre raised a relevant question about how QALYs are being used. Are there any areas in which people think that QALYs or QALY league tables have been misused in making decisions?

Peter Selby: One example, not of misuse but perhaps of undue prominence, might be in the Forrest report on breast cancer screening, in which there was an analysis based on QALYs (no doubt noted by those reading the report), yet little discussion of the technical merits of the QALY methodology which would have been appropriate in this context.[1]

Clive Smee: I agree that the Forrest report might have made such doubts clearer. There is a tendency to jump to the conclusion that QALYs are being used to make decisions. I hope that it is recognised that any piece of information, such as a cost-per-QALY, however calculated, will be only one component in informing decisions about resource allocation, which usually, at the end of the day, are based upon political judgements. The question then is whether QALYs should be provided as a piece of information, not whether decisions should be based on them, any more than just one piece of information is used when deciding where to build a road, for example.

The point made by Astrid Fletcher about aggregation of years of survival and quality of life seems related to similar problems in making decisions about resource allocation in other areas. There is always the issue of whether it is better to try to bring as many considerations as possible together into one number, or to present the managers and the politicians who make the ultimate judgements with all the pieces of information, leaving them to make the trade offs. This seems to me to go to the heart of the value, or lack of value, of the QALY. As Alan

Williams said, the unique contribution of the QALY is to try to bring together, into one number, length of survival and quality of life.

Douglas Black: John Grimley Evans would point out that QALYs are inherently unfair to the elderly. This is the general case of the problem of weighting. In the romantic days of health economics, Clive Smee's predecessor, David Pole, and I worked out indices of activity, taking in parameters such as outpatient attendances and inpatient days,[2] but what is then made of these in terms of a unitary measure depends entirely on the relative weighting given to each component. Given even hard primary data, there is still a conceptual problem in how those are weighted.

Alan Williams: The process of integrating life expectancy with quality of life tends to discriminate against people for whom the expectancy of life can be increased very little. Whether such discrimination is inequitable, however, requires another set of judgements. Discrimination itself is essential—this is the purpose of the exercise, and to prove that this has been done gets us nowhere. To prove that the discrimination is unfair, a whole set of other principles has to be adduced. There is nothing in the way in which items are added together in QALYs that requires it to be done so that a QALY is a QALY for everybody. If it is thought that a QALY for an old person should be valued higher than a QALY for a mother of young children, suitable adjustments can be made or, if the reverse, adjustments can be made the other way. Inequity is not inherent in QALYs.

Roy Carr-Hill: Clive Smee stated that the major issue about QALYs is whether managers and politicians should have an array of numbers before them or just one. I do not think this is the issue for democracy, but whether people can understand and react to the array of numbers. Managers cannot comprehend them, because they do not read the research reports. The public also needs to understand on what these numbers are based and how to reply to them. This issue of transparency requires that separate dimensions are measured separately and seen to be separate.

Clive Smee referred to the cost-benefit calculations in relation to building roads. This is a red herring. When there was discussion about the proposed outer ring road for London 25 years ago, I was part of a group which took the position that by far the most efficient and cost-effective policy, in terms of the criteria being used by the commission set up to study the problem, was to bring all cars into central London, crush them by bulldozers, and have perfect public transport—but this did not take into account the interests of car manufacturers, and so of course it did not happen. Resources have recently been put into planning where the rail link should go from the Channel Tunnel to London, and the route finally chosen was that which had been discarded on 'cost-benefit' grounds. The choice appears to have been heavily influenced by political considerations. It was known all along that the more direct route went through south London, but that the politicians there would not like it. The decision about the route was made on that elemental basis, and the study played only a symbolic role. This is a warning to people who feel that these indices may influence policy.

References

1. Forrest T. *Breast cancer screening*. Report to the Minister of Health by a working group chaired by Professor Sir Patrick Forrest. London: HMSO, 1986
2. Black DAK, Pole JD. Priorities in biomedical research: indices of burden. *British Journal of Preventive and Social Medicine* 1975; **29**: 222–7

4 | Are we satisfied with QALYs? What are the conceptual and empirical uncertainties and what must we do to make them more generally useful?

Martin Buxton

Director, Health Economics Research Group, Brunel University of West London

Introduction

For many years I have attempted to walk a tightrope between enthusiastic evangelism for the broad conceptual framework provided by quality-adjusted life years (QALYs) and cautious agnosticism about the ability adequately to operationalise the concept.[1,2] As a general concept, I have few reservations about QALYs: if rational decisions are to be made between alternatives within the health service, it is a tremendous advantage to be able to characterise the alternatives in terms of a single index measure of health benefit. Indeed, the current needs assessment/purchasing terminology of 'health gain' seems almost to presuppose the availability of such a measure. But, despite enthusiasm for the concept, I feel we need *at best* to treat current estimates with extreme caution as merely indicative of possible rela- tivities; *at worst*, there is little reason to believe that the estimates currently available are robust measures of the relative values placed by individuals or society on the combinations of quantity and quality of life they purport to reflect. Perhaps 'QALY league tables' should carry a government warning: 'These figures *may* seriously damage your perceptions of health'.

Thus, this paper starts from the standpoint that the aim of QALYs is laudable, the basic concept is appropriate and ethical, and QALYs potentially offer a powerful tool to assist in the determination of health service priorities, particularly when presented in relationship to cost. However, there is still a long list of major conceptual details and

empirical questions that need to be addressed critically before QALYs can be used with any confidence. The following questions seem to be the most important:
— is the descriptive system appropriate?
— is the valuation technique valid and reliable?
— is the value of the quality adjustment factor independent of the survival period or profile, or do values for health states reflect a complex interaction of the two?
— do the valuations adequately handle the attitudes to risk of the individuals or society?
— do the valuations adequately handle the individual or social time-preference for health benefits?
— are there, or should there be, factors other than the extent and quality of health gain that affect our valuations: eg age, sex, socio-economic status of the beneficiary or equity considerations?

There are a number of more technical reviews of such issues in the economic literature (eg ref. 3). This chapter attempts to address briefly each of these issues in an essentially non-technical manner, as a criticism of the current weaknesses of QALYs, and to indicate which issues need to be addressed to make them more useful. I conclude with a brief assessment of the implications of this for the current use of QALY estimates and 'cost per QALY league tables'.

The main issues

The appropriateness of the descriptive system

It will be clear from the previous chapters that there is no common agreement as to what constitutes an adequate descriptive system for this purpose. Health-related quality of life (which I believe is what needs to be described) is an imprecisely defined but undoubtedly multidimensional construct. Nevertheless, it is not surprising that a simple two-dimensional hierarchical matrix (from the original work of Rosser and colleagues) forms the basis for most of the existing QALY work in the UK.[4] It offers the not insubstantial practical advantage of requiring the valuation of only a small number (29) of health state combinations. However, the inadequacy of this matrix to reflect all the main dimensions of health-related quality of life is now, I believe, recognised by most people in the field, including Rosser herself, as shown by her presentation in this volume of a new/revised three-dimensional instrument (Chapter 7).

In general, the existing multidimensional instruments that might be argued to represent better the multidimensionality of health-related quality of life (for example, the Nottingham Health Profile (NHP), the Sickness Impact Profile or the US Medical Outcomes Study Short Form 36) have not been constructed to enable the classified health states to be firmly anchored into a scale from 0–1 (dead to full health). Theoretically, each combination health state (plus those involving full health) in terms of specific dimensions could be valued, but the NHP, for example, would in principle give rise to about 275,000 million combination states to be valued! Pragmatically, cautious attempts have been made to move from profile scores on such instruments to appropriate adjustment factors.[1,5] In practice, not all combinations are likely to occur: some dimensions appear to possess full or partial Guttman scale characteristics, and some combination responses would simply not arise.

If dimensions are hierarchically constructed, it may be possible to use multi-attribute scaling techniques, as has been tentatively suggested for the Euroqol instrument,[6] is now claimed for the Index of Health-Related Quality of Life (Chapter 7), and was previously developed by Torrance, Boyle and Horwood.[7] This technique considerably reduces the extent of the valuation procedure, but the independence of valuations for separate dimensions in any instrument, and the simple additivity or otherwise of the value for the combined multidimensional health states, need to be proven empirically and not simply assumed.

There has been a number of suggestions that the descriptive system underlying QALYs needs to be disease-specific.[8] Whilst it is easy to understand the desire to use descriptive systems that adequately and reliably distinguish health states experienced by particular patient groups, the whole purpose of QALYs is lost if the valuation systems are not consistent (viz, if an adjustment factor of 0.7 on one scale is not equivalent to an adjustment factor of 0.7 on another) or, in other words, if one of the scales does not possess all the characteristics required of it. Consistent scale values derived via a number of specific descriptive systems could well be an advantage. However, it needs to be recognised that QALY valuation systems are never likely to be so fine-grained that they can differentiate all the levels of health-related quality of life that would be distinguishable on specialised scales.

It is of course possible to bypass the descriptive process entirely, if valuations are sought only from patients who are experiencing (or have experienced) the specific health state in question. Direct valuation of individuals' own health using time trade off or standard gamble need not involve the use of any explicit descriptive system. This approach certainly has some conceptual advantages, but it is operationally unsatisfactory because it requires values to be measured afresh for each application of the QALY.

The validity and reliability of the method and process of valuation

Much attention has been paid in the literature to the competing merits of the various valuation methods (such as standard gamble, time trade off, magnitude estimation, category scaling, etc). This is not the place to rehearse the various claims and counterclaims, but it needs to be emphasised that there is relatively little comparative evidence from large-scale studies of the results of using different techniques for the same health state descriptors with the same or directly comparable respondents. The evidence currently available suggests, however, that the different techniques do *not* give the same results. Indeed, the results from any one technique may give very different results according to context, details of administration, framing effects, etc (eg Ref. 9).

Much more systematic evidence is needed on the relationship between value sets derived using the different techniques. There are some hints of broadly consistent relationships which, if confirmed, would at least enable cross-mapping of results.[10] This would be all the more useful if there could be common agreement about what represents the best technique, but such agreement is unlikely until some of the other questions have been addressed.

In the context of the much used 'Rosser values', there must be grave doubt that those valuations would be reproducible in other groups of respondents, by other researchers, or that they would be consistent with values for the same (imperfect) descriptive matrix obtained using, say, time trade off or standard gamble techniques. The research programme at the University of York has addressed these questions. There is now a real danger that this larger-scale work will produce very different results from the initial results on which so much of the work to date has been predicated in the UK.

There is little evidence of the stability of such values. Few thorough test-retest studies have been undertaken, and no longitudinal studies of whether and how individuals' values change over time. Results from some of our work at Brunel suggest that the first set of results from any individual should perhaps be ignored. In interviews at retest after 3–6 weeks, respondents have volunteered the observation that they believed their responses had changed. Prior to the first interview, they had not thought about values in this way, but the exercise had led to subsequent reflection.[11] However posed, the valuation task is not one with which the average respondent will have had any previous experience or to which he will be likely to have given prior consideration.

The relationship of health state values to their duration, sequence or profile

The commonly adopted two-step process of first applying predetermined values for health states as constants independent of the length of the period of time to which they apply, and then of summing the independently calculated values of these periods to give the value for a sequence of different health states begs two important questions at least. First, the initial values for the health states may have depended on the time period specified in the original valuation task. A number of studies have suggested that such values will vary with the time period considered (see Ref. 12). There is no basis (except convenience) for assuming a constant proportional trade off between length of life and health status.[3] Thus, the original values obtained may be duration-dependent, but this is ignored because they are applied to diverse periods of health without adjustment. It is worrying that values obtained relating typically to a period of one year may also be applied both to brief acute episodes of a few days and to chronic states of many years. Furthermore, values may be dependent on the sequence of health states, and it may strictly be necessary to obtain values for each such lifetime sequence. This perspective has been taken up in the work of Mehrez and Gafni in estimating what they distinguish as 'healthy-year equivalents',[13] an approach which has been followed by Richardson.[14] To what extent such a conceptual refinement is empirically important requires further evidence, although Mehrez and Gafni illustrate their argument with examples where values might indeed differ.

Handling of risk

Different valuation techniques handle risk differently, and it is one factor that might help to determine the preferred technique. Standard gamble involves explicit risk, and the resultant values are influenced by the respondents' attitudes to risk. It has been well documented that the framing of questions involving risk is critical, and even doctors view a 5% mortality rate differently from a 95% survival rate.[15]

The time trade off approach offers certain (viz, riskless) choices, and appears to avoid the problem, although respondents may not believe in a riskless choice and still incorporate in their response an assumed risk. Similarly, the Rosser values, calculated by a direct ratio technique, are seemingly risk-neutral. However, it is not clear, to me at least, whether or not non-neutral attitudes to risk should be incorporated into QALY calculations.

The handling of time preference

In obtaining values, just as the standard gamble is 'contaminated' by the respondent's attitude to risk, so time trade off is 'contaminated' by time preference and implicit discounting. In economic evaluation, the issue of discounting tends to receive little attention, with economists often preferring to discourage wide discussion of a 'technical' issue. But discounting and the choice of discount rate matter, and it is important accurately to reflect the time preference of individuals or society for health benefits. The most common approach is to discount health benefits at the same rate as costs for 'consistency'.[16] For example, discounting of benefits reduces the attractiveness of interventions that have the characteristic of an investment, for example, surgical as compared to medical interventions, or preventive measures as compared to subsequent treatment of disease. The evidence on the time preference of individuals for health benefits is limited and conflicting.[17] But there are good arguments to suggest that health benefits such as QALYs, expressed in non-monetary terms, should be discounted at a lower rate than costs, or even at a zero discount rate.[18]

The relevance of other factors

The basic tenet of the QALY approach is that a year of full-quality health, or its equivalent in a greater number of years of health of poorer quality, is regarded as of equal value, irrespective of other characteristics of the beneficiary. My view is that this appears to be a defensible egalitarian position. However, it may be that individuals or society take, or should take, certain other factors into account, in particular perhaps the stage in an individual's life cycle and/or his family responsibilities. Work undertaken at York suggests that a sample of the general population values health most highly in children and in those bringing up children.[19]

The calculus of QALYs treats a gain of 20 QALYs to one individual as of equal value to a gain of one QALY to 20 individuals, or of 0.01 QALYs to 2,000 individuals. I suspect this is not how the National Health Service behaves, or probably how society expects it to behave. Do some additional equity considerations need to be built into QALY calculations?[20]

Whose values of health should count? This question has to be answered politically. Society, or politicians on its behalf, has to decide, rather than economists or evaluators of health services. At this stage, good evidence is needed regarding whether and to what extent values differ between different groups and, if they do vary, in what consistent ways. The empirical implications of the choice as to whose values can then be assessed.

Conclusions

It is important to make a number of points after such a list of criticisms, questions and uncertainties: first to acknowledge that all the matters I have raised are well-known to those working in the field, and many people are trying to undertake the difficult empirical research that is required if they are to be positively addressed. Secondly, to recognise that any modelling of such a complex reality as the nature and value of health states following health care interventions must *necessarily* involve some abstraction and simplification, and any conceptualisation that attempts to incorporate this complexity into one index value must necessarily lose some of the detail. The real question is whether there are oversimplifications or assumptions that distort the reality and lead to misleading results. At this stage, I believe there is not enough evidence to satisfy critics on these points. A research agenda is needed that will enable the basic conceptual framework to be made operational from a much stronger empirical justification, and also a willingness to adapt the detailed QALY methods to reflect the best evidence that can be obtained.

It is also important to remember that cost per QALY league tables involve many problems in addition to those addressed here, which all relate essentially to the quality adjustment factor or the alternative methods for valuing health states. There is great uncertainty surrounding other elements of the calculus, such as the cost estimates or the expected survival. There seems to be an unwarranted assumption that these estimates are unchanging over time. Average and marginal values need to be distinguished clearly. Also, the league tables are best characterised by the enormity of the range of interventions which are totally excluded because there are no data on them.

What then is a justifiable position to adopt at this stage? The concept should certainly be promulgated as a 'heuristic approach'. There is very little by way of alternative to assist in rational resource allocation in the health service—but it should be remembered that the current QALY values and league tables may be writ in wax rather than stone!

References

1. O'Brien BJ, Buxton MJ, Ferguson B. Measuring the effectiveness of heart transplant programmes: quality of life data and their relationship to survival analysis. *Journal of Chronic Diseases* (suppl 1) 1987; **40**: 137–53S

2. Buxton MJ. The economic evaluation of high technology medicine: the case of heart transplants. In: Williams A, ed. *Health and economics*. Basingstoke: Macmillan, 1987

3. Loomes G, McKenzie L. The use of QALYs in health care decision making. *Social Science and Medicine* 1989; **28**: 299–308

4. Kind P, Rosser R, Williams A. Valuation of quality of life: some psychometric evidence. In: Jones-Lee MW, ed. *The value of life and safety*. Amsterdam: North Holland, 1982

5. Ferguson B, Buxton MJ. Analysing Nottingham Health Profile data: identifying common response patterns. *Health Economics Research Group Discussion Paper no. 3*. Uxbridge: Brunel University, 1986

6. Euroqol Group. Euroqol© — a new facility for the measurement of health-related quality of life. *Health Policy* 1990; **16**: 199–208

7. Torrance GW, Boyle MH, Horwood SP. Application of multi-attribute utility theory to measure social preferences for health states. *Operations Research* 1982; **30**: 1043–69

8. Donaldson C, Atkinson A, Bond J, Wright K. Should QALYs be programme-specific? *Journal of Health Economics* 1988; **7**: 239–57

9. Llewellyn-Thomas H, Sutherland HJ, Tibshirani R, Ciampi A, Till JE, Boyd NF. Describing health states: methodological issues in obtaining values for health states. *Medical Care* 1984; **22**: 543–52

10. Buxton MJ, Ashby J. The time trade off approach to health state valuation. In: Teeling-Smith G, ed. *Measuring health: a practical guide*. Chichester: John Wiley & Sons, 1988

11. Buxton MJ, Ashby J, O'Hanlon M. Alternative methods of valuing health states: a comparative analysis based on an empirical study using the time trade off approach in relation to health states one year after treatment for breast cancer. *HERG Discussion Paper no. 2*. Brunel University, 1986

12. Torrance GW. Measurement of health state activities for economic appraisal: a review. *Journal of Health Economics* 1986; **5**: 1–30

13. Mehrez A, Gafni A. Quality-adjusted life years, utility theory, and healthy-years equivalents. *Medical Decision Making* 1989; **9**: 142–9

14. Richardson J. Cost utility analyses: what should be measured — utility, value or healthy-year equivalents? *NHMRC National Centre for Health Program Evaluation Working Paper no. 5*. 1990. National Health and Medical Research Council, Fairfield, Victoria, Australia

15. O'Brien BJ. *What are my chances doctor? — a review of clinical risks*. London: Office of Health Economics, 1986

16. Weinstein MC, Stason WB. Foundations of cost-effectiveness analysis for health and medical practices. *New England Journal of Medicine* 1977; **296**: 716–21

17. Lipscomb J. Time preference for health in cost-effectiveness analysis. *Medical Care* 1989; **27**: S233–53.

18. Parsonage M, Neuburger J. Discounting and health benefits. *Health Economics* 1992; **1**: 71–9

19. Wright SJ. Age, sex and health: a summary of the findings from the York Health Evaluation Survey. *Centre for Health Economics Discussion Paper 15*. York: University of York, 1986.

20. Wagstaff A. QALYs and the equity-efficiency trade off. *Journal of Health Economics* 1991; **10**: 21–41

DISCUSSION

Ian Russell: I agree with Martin Buxton that the aims of what he calls QALYs, but what should perhaps be called health status-adjusted life years, are laudable and that the basic concept is appropriate and ethical. I also agree that QALYs have the potential to help in setting health service priorities, and that the two-stage method of estimating health status, first describing and then valuing the states, suffers from many practical problems. However, I believe he has omitted the biggest problem of all in operationalising QALYs: that of estimating the frequency distribution of the stream of descriptive states suffered by the population of patients under review. To take the example of coronary artery bypass grafting, it is difficult enough to estimate the successive states suffered by a typical patient undergoing coronary artery bypass graft, and even more difficult to estimate the wide range of experiences of all such potential patients. Alan Williams' paper on the economics of coronary artery bypass grafting, although pioneering and influential, did not address the question of what happens to this population.[1]

I want to offer an alternative method of estimating health status, and to suggest that it overcomes many of Martin Buxton's six problems and even goes some way to tackling the additional problem that I have mentioned. This is the time trade off approach, but not the version tested and discussed by Martin Buxton in which respondents are asked what part of their remaining life expectancy they would trade for good health over that lifetime which, as he pointed out, is contaminated by time preference. It is instead Ken Buckingham's proposal that respondents should be asked what part of the next 24 hours they would trade in the form of additional sleep, which they forgo, for good health over those 24 hours—changing the time scale of time trade off, so that it is no longer a lifetime calculation but a 24-hour calculation. It has immediately to be acknowledged that the question has to be worded very carefully to avoid problems with insomnia and so on. Buckingham and colleagues in the Health Service's Research Unit have now put this question to more than 2,000 respondents, including over 800 asthma outpatients interviewed at home, with a response rate of over 90%. Random samples of the population of Aberdeen have also been interviewed, some 70% of whom responded to the question in the form of a postal questionnaire.

These studies suggest that the approach is both feasible and valid, as judged by high correlation with other measures of health outcome, notably the short form of the RAND medical outcome survey instrument, the SF36.[2] Instead of discussing further the daily time trade off approach at this stage, it may be assessed against the six practical problems listed in Martin Buxton's paper:

The appropriateness of the descriptive system: time trade off is a direct or one-stage method of valuing health, so there is no need for an underlying descriptive system, which in itself creates much of the arguments already raised. The daily time trade off approach has proved operationally satisfactory.

The validity and reliability of the valuation method and process: it is hoped that it will soon be possible to respond to Martin Buxton's call for comparative evidence from large-scale studies using different techniques in surveys of about 2,000 people. The valuation task facing the average respondent is tackled frequently in deciding when to go to bed and when to get up.

The relationship of health state values to their duration, sequence or profile: time trade off is a direct method of valuing health, so it can bypass the problem that a length of time spent in a given state may affect the value of that state. If necessary, there can be more frequent sampling.

The handling of risk: the time trade off approach appears to offer riskless choices, as Martin Buxton stated, but it would be prudent at some time in the future also to address this issue, and to test it in a sample of in-depth interviews.

The handling of time preference: the daily time trade off approach is believed to avoid the problem of implicit discounting by offering respondents, at least by implication, the opportunity to re-assess their trade off decision day by day. Perhaps more importantly, given the earlier discussion, it offers respondents the opportunity to trade time for health—an opportunity which some contributors to this book seem to want to deny them.

The relevance of other factors: we also agree with Martin Buxton about the need to investigate the influence of other factors, and are currently pursuing this, especially in our studies of the general public.

Variation among patients: the finding that health valuations elicited by the daily time trade off approach are highly correlated with the responses to the SF36 offers a means of tackling the additional problem of incorporating variation between patients into the QALY calculus. In effect, it has been shown that daily time trade off can be used to derive health values directly from the SF36. Furthermore, colleagues in the USA have suggested, with a fair amount of empirical evidence, that SF36 can be administered at regular intervals as a means of estimating health gain within a population. Thus, if daily time trade off is combined with SF36 it may be possible to derive a method of valuing health gain over entire populations—a method that would overcome many of Martin Buxton's six problems.

Clive Smee: It might not be profitable to discuss further whether Ian Russell's approach may be an answer to some of our problems without having been able to study the proposals first, but at least there is agreement between him and Martin Buxton that until now there have been these major problems.

Alan Williams: The problems identified by Martin Buxton are on the agenda, and I have no difficulty in accepting everything he says. It is only money and time that prevent us proceeding with them. However, there will still be a problem if people use different quality of life measures in every separate field because it will be impossible to make comparisons between the valuations of health states associated with different disorders.

References

1. Williams A. The economics of coronary bypass grafting. *British Medical Journal* 1991; **291**: 325–9
2. SF36. US Medical Outcomes Study Short Form 36

5 | Are QALYs going to be useful to me as a purchaser of health services?

Paul Walker
Director of Public Health, Norwich District Health Authority

Introduction

As a public health physician, I shall give the purchaser's perspective on quality-adjusted life years (QALYs), in particular their use in determining health and health care priorities. Although I have been interested in QALYs for a long time, both as a district general manager and, more recently, as a public health physician in the new internal market, I have found them to be more useful as a conceptual framework for communicating with fellow senior officers and health authority members than as a practical day-to-day tool. Over the last two years I have used the instrument of the annual report as a means to inform and educate my colleagues on the concept of QALYs as the best approximation to a common calculus or language for health. It would be wrong to say that my colleagues are fully converted to the concept, but I believe they are well on the way. I have quoted a range of QALY costs in my annual report, but it is fair to say that, at a conscious level at least, no decisions have been made by my health authority solely, or even predominantly, on the basis of QALY scores.

The conceptual framework for health

One of the difficulties in discussing the role of health authorities and how they make decisions is that, as far as I am aware, no coherent attempt has been made to define the conceptual framework and language for health against which to assess their decision-making role. There is a need to define some of the basic concepts. I have used the annual report, amongst other things, as a tool for conceptual development. Table 1 illustrates the relevant section from my 1990 annual report which sets the scene, as it were, on the direction of thinking in the Norwich Health Authority.

The framework introduces the three terms, healthiness, health state

53

Table 1. Conceptual framework for health.[1]

Determinants	Entity	Impacts
Life-style		Distress
Environment		Disability
Human biology	Disease	Quality of life
Health care organisation		Premature mortality
Healthiness	*Health state*	*Health status (Healthfulness)*

and health status, relating to the determinants of health, the disease entity and the impacts of disease, respectively. Healthfulness is another term sometimes used for health status. I consider that *health state* represents the present health state of an individual, as distinct from his *health status* which is a longer-term attribute. Health state is akin to the economist's concept of 'flow', whereas health status is akin to 'stock'.

The above framework is useful only to the extent that it helps identify health promoting and protecting interventions by the health authority and other health agencies. The range of such interventions includes the following:

— *Prevention of disease* through changes in life-style, manipulation of the environment, and alteration of human biology where possible. The scope for this type of intervention is broad, and involves many agencies in addition to the health care agencies: for example, environmental health, housing and social services departments, the Health and Safety Executive, and so on.

— *Cure* or *control* of established disease through the application of modern therapeutic technology. This is an almost exclusive preserve of health care.

— *Relief of distress* through the application of a variety of technologies, including drugs and counselling. This is largely the responsibility of health care.

— *Reduction in disability/handicap* through the restoration of lost function where possible, and compensation for it where restoration is not possible. These interventions are, in part, the responsibility of health care, but to a significant degree also the responsibility of other agencies such as social services and housing.

— *Improvement in quality of life* through a mixture of interventions relating particularly to the relief of distress and the reduction in disability as outlined above. These interventions are the responsibility of health care and also of other organisations such as social services and housing.

— *Avoidance of premature mortality* through the application of appropriate resuscitation and treatment technologies. These interventions are the exclusive preserve of health care.

Promoting and protecting the public health therefore necessarily involve the following:
— preventing preventable disease;
— curing curable established disease and, where this is not possible, controlling controllable disease;
— relieving relievable distress resulting from disease;
— restoring and compensating for disability resulting from disease;
— avoiding avoidable premature mortality resulting from disease.

Not all aspects of health are changeable in the present state of knowledge, or under currently acceptable ethical frameworks. Hence the various states of health, ie healthiness, health state and health status, can be seen as either mutable or non-mutable. Where an aspect of health is mutable, the appropriate change may be achieved through an intervention by health care services, or possibly social services where it is possible to contract for the appropriate intervention. Alternatively, the required intervention may have to come from another agency outside the contracting domain through the application by the health authority of influence and leadership. Thus, there are the concepts of *contractables* and *influenceables* — and perhaps a third category of *non-contractable/influenceables!*[1]

QALYs and the role of the health authority

Broadly speaking, I see the role of the health authority as the application of the utilitarian ethic to health and social care constrained by considerations of equity and of affirmative action. This role is manifest in the making of explicit choices in the form of the authority's purchasing, joint purchasing and intersectoral plans.

The concept of the QALY is applicable at the purchasing and intersectoral planning levels, but may not be so applicable in the area of joint purchasing with, for example, social services. In Norfolk, an attempt has been made to define a health and social care needs assessment framework which will define the contributions of the health service, social services and other agencies, such as housing, to health and social care in those areas where they clearly interrelate. The concept of handicap has been selected as the link between the health service and other agencies. 'Handicap' is used here in the sense defined by Wood as part of an overall framework comprising disease/disorder, impairment, disability and handicap.[2] The relationship between these concepts is shown in Fig. 1.

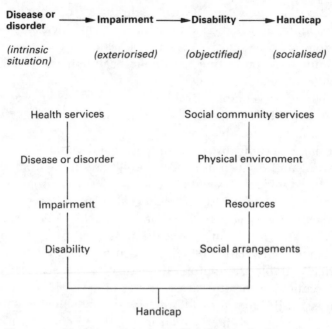

Fig. 1. *Two ways of looking at the genesis of handicap or disadvantage.*

The concept of handicap used in this way focuses attention on social roles rather than on function. This raises a question about the possible value of QALYs in the area of joint purchasing of health and social care because, by definition, QALYs focus on disability rather than on handicap. Do QALYs need to be redefined in terms of handicap rather than disability? If so, is the resulting Mark II QALY to be used only in the joint purchasing domain, or should it replace the Mark I QALY in all health and social care? It is my view that the concept of handicap based on social roles is more powerful than that based on disability.

Practical application of QALYs by the health authority

At a more practical level, I am interested in using QALY scores in the following areas:
— at the level of individual interventions;
— at the service level;
— at the population level;
— in the context of waiting lists.
   Traditionally, QALYs have been applied at the level of individual interventions. In the new contracting environment, where contracts for service will be increasingly specified in terms of individual inter-

ventions, this will become an important area for the application of QALYs in seeking to achieve the best possible added value to the public health from the contracting process.

On the basis of the QALY/cost scores quoted by Bryan *et al.* in 1988, contracts in Norwich for 1992–93 will seek to increase the number of hip replacements and to increase substantially the number of kidney transplants for patients with end-stage renal failure in the expectation of substantially reducing the financial burden of home and hospital haemodialysis.

At a higher level of aggregation, health authorities are interested in trying to optimise their investment strategies in different blocks of health care, such as general acute services, mental health, mental handicap, care of the elderly and prevention of illness. Although there are many other considerations apart from QALYs in defining such a strategy, it is my view that decisions in this area would be 'better' if they were adequately informed by considerations of cost-utility such as QALY scores.

Public health physicians are of course interested in relating health care services to the needs of populations, in particular in measuring the health of their populations. Traditionally, suitably standardised mortality measures, such as standardised mortality ratios (SMRs), have been used, on the basis of which my health district is probably the healthiest in the UK. I believe that the QALY concept should start to be applied to population health, so that due weight can be given to the quality of life of populations—which, there is reason to believe, might be rather less in my health district than elsewhere. In my next annual report I hope to derive a population QALY measure both from local mortality data and from specific health status and health evaluation data obtained locally in a population survey which used the Euroqol© questionnaire.

In our health district, attempts are being made to apply public health concepts to waiting lists. We are keen to apply some of the methods piloted by Williams and Gudex at Guy's Hospital on our notoriously long waiting list.[3] The aim is to devise referral protocols for the various surgical specialties using available QALY data, to ensure both that the surgical capability is used to best QALY effect and that patients with low QALY impact conditions cease to be referred through normal referral channels.

The use of QALYs in purchasing and intersectoral plans

The use of the QALY concept to define purchasing and intersectoral strategies, rather than as a broad educational tool on health, requires much more information on QALYs than currently exists. It is frustrating for a public health physician to find how relatively few QALY scores are available. Having included the Bryan *et al.* selection in my 1990 report, I have tried to compile a comprehensive list for my latest annual report and have found it very difficult. QALY scores are needed not only for all significant health care interventions, but almost certainly also stratified by age and sex. The QALY score for an inguinal herniorrhaphy clearly will be different for a 35-year-old man to that for a 65-year-old and the difference needs to be known. As indicated above, the use of QALYs also needs to be developed at the service level to help define inter-service strategy. Investment in both mental handicap and general acute services, for example, needs to be looked at in the same terms — and preferably in QALY terms. This raises important problematic issues about measures of quality of life of people with severe learning disabilities.

The appropriate unit for health measurement

Another issue looming increasingly large in my thinking on public health is the appropriate unit for health measurement. Traditionally, the health of populations has been thought of as the sum of the health of individuals, considered as individuals. Looking at the quality of life of patients with mental illness and/or physical disability, the effect on their immediate carers of the health of individual patients is striking. This raises the need to look at the health of such social units rather than at the health of patients individually.

Conclusions

QALYs may not be the universal calculus of health care, and using them will not result in the depoliticisation of setting priorities for health care. However, they represent, I believe, an important stage in the development both of our thinking about health status and of a common language for expressing health states. Using QALYs would also result in a clearer delineation of those elements of setting priorities which are strictly factual, based upon scientific research, and those which are clearly political or ethical. Such an explicit factorisation of decision making in health would be highly desirable.

References

1. *Annual Report of the Director of Public Health to Norwich Health Authority,* 1990

2. World Health Organisation. *International classification of impairments, disabilities and handicaps*. Geneva: WHO, 1980
3. Williams A, Gudex C. *Health Trends* 1990; **22**(3)

DISCUSSION

Christopher Pollitt: Some of the earlier discussions have suggested only two rather extreme scenarios: the first, in which doctors, health care managers and politicians resolutely ignore QALY-type measures and, at the other extreme, these measures are so seductive that people follow them blindly without fully understanding them and arrive at inappropriate decisions. Paul Walker has made it clear that there are positions between those two extremes—surely this is the territory in which we will all operate over the next few years.

Although QALYs are not designed to be political, they inevitably are in the sense that any tool which can be used for resource allocation is bound to be political. Perhaps, though, they are political in an extra sense in the health care world because they appear to provide a measure of the utility of interventions, but one which, unlike others, is not overwhelmingly owned by the medical profession. QALYs seem to have been invented, at least in part, by economists, and also appear to be devices which can be understood—or perhaps misunderstood—as easily by managers as by doctors. This is an important feature not to lose sight of because the boundaries of authority and responsibility between managers and doctors in the health service are moving. Paul Walker writes that, at a conscious level at least, no decisions have been made by his health authority solely, or even predominantly, on the basis of QALY scores—but why not?

There are at least three possible answers:
— he could not get the data;
— the people taking the decisions did not trust the method;
— there was some form of self-interested resistance, even if the data were available and the method understood and tolerably robust.

It would be interesting to know which of these or other reasons has produced the situation in which the information is beginning to be available but is apparently not in any way dominating health authority decisions. If there is resistance to the introduction of QALY measures, it is important to understand its nature.

Paul Walker discussed the possible value of QALYs in joint purchasing and whether some kind of measure of social roles should be included. If the concept of distress is once admitted to the measurement of the quality of life, most non-specialists would find it artificial to exclude from that concept the distress experienced on being deprived, or partly deprived, of our most important social relationships, or when their quality is strikingly reduced. I believe that QALYs need to be redefined, in order to include a broader concept than was possible originally. (This question is also dealt with by Howard Glennerster in Chapter 11.)

Paul Walker refers to 'depoliticisation'. If there is anything to transparency, it is certainly not depoliticisation. Initially, transparency in this, as in many other areas, is almost bound to lead to political excitement—not necessarily and not exclusively party political excitement—but to politicise decisions is not necessarily to democratise them, and there is a whole series of further considerations between transparency and democracy.

Finally, I would like to pose directly two questions which Paul Walker implicitly poses. The first concerns the use of QALYs. He has discussed them partly in terms that they may help a health authority to discriminate between different types of intervention. Can he see a time when they may help discriminate between different providers, so that he might start to move contracts because of information indicating a substantial difference between the quality of care given by two providers? Secondly, a key question is how a manager in a health authority can contribute to the process of educating the public, the managers, and the doctors—all the people involved in health care decision making—so that some understanding of the nature of these instruments begins to spread. I would be interested to hear whether he thinks some slightly more aggressive or expansive attempt to educate this audience would be possible.

Paul Walker: The general issue of whether to select providers of care on the basis of cost and quality is difficult in Norfolk because there are monopoly suppliers in different sectors of care. However, the short answer is yes, in principle. By using the leverage of the contracting process, information may be obtained about outcomes. We want to choose on issues of quality—whatever that is, and however it is measured.

Linda Lamont: If the public are to be involved in setting priorities— and it is important that they are—it is crucial to consider how to explain the QALY concept to them. The experts must think about how to do this in a simple way. If we are talking about resource allocation and setting priorities, we cannot afford to wait another decade while people decide what QALYs mean.

Astrid Fletcher: Paul Walker said that the public should be asked to participate in setting priorities by valuing states of health, but how I as an individual might value a state of health and how I might decide that resources should be spent may not be the same. It is being assumed that the valuation of health states implies decisions by people about how money should be spent.

Alan Williams: When we asked people about their views on the value of different health states and what views they thought the NHS should have, there was no significant difference between the answers.

Howard Glennerster: I am keen to try to explain measures of quality of life (of which there may be several) to the general public, but it is much more difficult to convince people that QALYs are useful. From his experience of talking to members of a health authority, did Paul Walker find in practice that the two concepts were considered synonymous?

Anthony Hopkins: I am sure that quality of life measures and QALYs should not be confused—they have different dimensions, the second including time. It is scientifically invalid to talk interchangeably about different dimensions.

Paul Walker: Our health authority did not have a big debate about QALYs. One of the strengths of QALYs for members of health authorities is that it avoids them having to think about a range of different ways of measuring quality of life.

Howard Glennerster: That is the problem: it is what I do want them to think about. That remark makes the whole point about transparency.

Paul Walker: We did not go through the interim phase of asking what is meant by quality of life, discussing the various instruments and how to get from there to QALYs. I made the leap straight to QALYs. It seemed to be a simplifying concept for them, which I think they understood.

Lesley Fallowfield: The use of the terms 'quality of life' and 'QALY' is more than just a question of semantics. There is a clear distinction between the sort of quality of life measures I use routinely in my work and those that tend to be used for the generation of QALYs. I take issue with Paul Walker that the problem is simple. If it appears so simple to him, he may be missing points that need to be explored further because the issues about quality of life and resource allocation are complex.

As a psychologist, I also have deep concerns about this notion that a judgement made at one point in time is a fixture upon which we can rely. My experience of working with patients, or with people who become patients, who then either are in a state of chronic ill health or become cured, is their great ability to adjust and cope with wide-ranging changes in their health state over time. Despite huge functional impairments resulting from disease, many people nevertheless maintain a good quality of life. If people in their well state are asked to make these sorts of trade off judgements, the data are of interest but do not relate to the judgements they would make in a changing or changed state when rendered sick by disease or treatment.

The debate is starting to confuse the issues related to the difference between quality of life assessment and the sort of data that can be incorporated into QALY assessments. If the issues are not properly worked out yet, it is better to continue muddling along in the way to which we are accustomed.

Roy Carr-Hill: There are dangers in the attraction of simple numbers—which may mask all kinds of things. There is an increasing tendency for numbers to be used in organisations and management, but they must be used with care. To take the example of resource allocation to different geographical regions, the only measure that has proved sufficiently robust is SMRs. It would be a waste of money to go down a road where neither the concept nor the principles of construction of these measures is clear.

Sally Macintyre: I think that health authority members and the public might be concerned about a measure focusing only on the individual patient. In allocating resources, carers and the knock-on effects of treatments have also to be considered. Paul Walker's authority should discuss the possibility of having some sort of QALY that takes into account the impact on other individuals in the social environment, in particular parents and those caring for elderly or disabled people, as well as the target individual.

6 | Do we need measures other than QALYs?

Sonja Hunt and Stephen McKenna

Senior Consultants, Galen Research & Consultancy, West Didsbury, Manchester

Introduction

The term 'quality of life' is relatively new in the field of health, having appeared in the literature less than 20 years ago. Since then, its use has grown exponentially, fuelled by the increasing need to evaluate medical and other procedures. However, the rush to measurement has resulted in a number of undesirable side-effects:

1. There has been a failure to reach an agreed definition of 'quality of life', giving rise to a confusing diversity of indicators ranging from, for example, the number of bowel movements[1] to whole batteries of physical and psychological tests.[2]
2. No conceptual basis or theoretical model has been developed which links quality of life to health-related and medical procedures and interventions.
3. Instruments have been adopted which were never intended to measure 'quality of life'.
4. There has been a failure to recognise and examine the social basis of definitions and measurement.
5. The concepts of 'quality of life' and 'quality of care' have tended to be used interchangeably.

Medical and economic approaches to quality of life

The introduction of quality-adjusted life years (QALYs)[3] illustrates most of these points, and exemplifies the adoption of particular methods of evaluation which rest upon a medical model of human health and an economic approach to the assessment of interventions. This has created an uneasy alliance which has given birth to some strange offspring. The medical model assumes that individual treatment pursued on a biochemical-surgical basis is the best way to tackle health problems. In this model, the doctor (as professional) is the best judge of both treatment and outcome. The discipline of health economics, on the other hand, is less concerned with individuals and more orientated towards a macro view of group phenomena in society at large.

These two extremes leave little room for the personal preferences of the patient, the social construction of illness or the contextual aspects of recovery. QALYs imply a mechanistic view of human existence, and cannot encompass the fact that the content of health services is not solely that patients *are* treated, but the *way* they are treated, by whom, in what circumstances, in what surroundings and with what sequelae.

Where social scientists have been involved in the measurement of health they have tended to adopt a Parsonian definition of health as the optimal capacity of an individual for the performance of roles and tasks for which he or she has been socialised.[4]

This functional focus fits well with a medical model which can incorporate such simple indicators of recovery as return to work. However, questions about the nature of the work, whether work is a valued activity, the effect of return to work on other important activities, or the availability of work, do not fit so well within the functional approach. Economists' notions of cost/utility have the same functional bias, although they recognise that at present return to work has little economic value in the UK.

Both medicine and economics are inclined to adopt the same 'top down' perspective of the 'expert'. Where patients are consulted they are often required to express themselves in the language of professionals and to address the concerns of the professionals rather than their own. For example, some self-completed questionnaires are assumed to reflect matters of importance to the patient, when they are in reality asking the patient about matters of interest to the clinician. The use of techniques such as 'standard gamble' or 'time trade off' by econometricians to elicit lay preferences requires lay people to adopt professional artifices which have little meaning in the real world of pain and hope.

In general, neither doctors nor economists can be expected to have expertise in judgements on quality of life since they have received relevant training neither in human social psychology nor in the appropriate techniques of design and measurement. This is reflected, unfortunately, in the many poor 'quality of life' studies, which often have no control groups, inappropriate outcome measures and faulty interpretation of results.

The evaluation of the experience and values of patients lies in a very different domain from that of clinical assessment or cost-effectiveness, where the criteria for measurement are much clearer even if the methods are not always valid.

The prevailing emphasis on function as a focus for external evaluation preserves the supremacy of the health professional as observer. This emphasis has been contrasted by Kelman with the experiential evaluation, which represents the inner experience of the person.[5] An accumulating body of research from medical sociology, and also trends in health policy towards a more consumer-led service, are moving evaluative strategies slowly from a professional towards a lay orientation. An important thread running through this has been a series of studies which show discrepancies between lay and professional judgements on several important parameters which govern the need for resources, both financial and human, in the health services.

Quality-adjusted life years (QALYs)

In Britain, the calculation of QALYs has been based largely upon the disability/distress matrix of Rosser.[6,7] Judgements about disability are founded in an observed lack of function and mobility in the patient, and were ranked by doctors or other health service personnel on a scale from none to unconsciousness and death. Distress is ranked in four categories: none, mild, moderate and severe. However, these categories are not defined. Furthermore, it is unclear whether the judgement of distress is obtained by asking the patient or from an external observer. There has been some criticism in the literature both of the methods and of the ethics of the QALY approach.[8-11] Clearly, this matrix is not a measure of health-related quality of life, but an estimate of disability and distress growing out of confused conceptual roots.

Recent attempts to operationalise the QALY have emerged in the form of the QALY Toolkit[12] and the Euroqol.[13] However, the content of these 'measures' appears arbitrary: there is no evidence of validity or reliability of the content, and some items will not apply to all potential respondents, thus raising problems of non-applicability and missing values. Moreover, the content does not take into account the tendency of patients with long-standing chronic conditions to adapt and adjust their lives to the illness (see Lesley Fallowfield's contribution to the Discussion in Chapter 5). Thus, a response to an enquiry as to whether state of health is affecting, say, social activities will be misleading if they have already been adjusted to individual capacity.

Above all, these instruments are not 'user-friendly', and the content does not take into account the concerns of patients, but rather is based upon the notions that professionals have about patients. In a recent study comparing a number of questionnaires for use with people suffering from epilepsy, only half of 40 patients were able to complete the disability section of the QALY toolkit, and only four fully understood the distress section. The visual analogue scale caused many problems, since patients were unclear about the nature of the task, and even when they did mark the line, subsequent questioning indicated that similar loci had a different meaning for different patients.[14] These problems were not a consequence of the mental or physical state of the patients who were able to complete other measures with greater ease.

Nevertheless, a two-dimensional outcome measure has advantages for setting priorities and considerations of cost in the health service, but for such a measure to be used it must be of high quality and provide information to decision makers which is both valid and reliable. If this is not achieved, there is no reason to believe that it will result in correct decisions being made. The measurement of disability and distress should build on the progress in health measurement made in the last 20 years rather than opting for simplistic techniques of poor quality. For example, the measurement of disability cannot consist of a few 'representative' questions because disability is not a single concept. The International Classification of Impairments, Disabilities and Handicaps (ICIDH) lists nine types of disability: behaviour, communication, personal care, locomotor, body disposition, dexterity, situational, particular skills and other activity restrictions.[15] Unless each of these is to be measured by the instrument, some form of summary concept must be used, the best of which, we would argue, is the physical independence/handicap dimension proposed by the ICIDH.

The value of using a measure of independence (or conversely, dependency) is that it has greater relevance to cost and the use of resources in the health service. Level of dependence reflects the impact of all the impairments and disabilities of the patient, as well as the resources available to ameliorate them. An individual may be quite severely disabled and yet not constitute a drain on resources, since he or she is able to maintain independence. Furthermore, the goal of a wide range of treatments and care options is to return a patient to independent status, or to maintain him in his present state as long as possible. This has particular relevance for the NHS and Community Care Act and the purchasing of health services. Moreover, it is possible for a person to be either more or less independent than his level of disability might suggest to an observer. Therefore, dependency is the suitable companion to distress for locating individuals on the QALY matrix. We are currently developing a patient-completed measure of dependency to accompany a new measure of distress.

The limitations of QALYs as an aid to decision making in the National Health Service (NHS)

Even if it were possible to provide valid and reliable QALY values as a basis for decision making in the health service, several difficulties would remain:

1. QALYs are unlikely to be sufficiently sensitive for the evaluation of efficacy in some situations, for example when assessing differences between two competing but essentially similar pharmaceutical products.
2. QALYs cannot cope well with less severe health problems where distress and disability or dependency are less relevant.
3. Preventive strategies, initiatives to promote health and the assessment of health needs require very different forms of assessment.
4. Interventions to halt or alter the natural history of illness, for example, in relation to the treatment of diabetes, will require more subtle and multidimensional scales.
5. Mental suffering, whether or not amounting to mental illness, constitutes a significant proportion of help-seeking within the NHS. Presently available measures of the QALY type are inappropriate. Indeed, emotional problems have been all but totally ignored in the assessment of the impact of treatments on 'quality of life', however defined.
6. Such an index is of little use in obtaining information about carers or significant others in the treatment process.
7. The implications of dependency and distress differ for different groups and individuals according to their responsibilities and the context of their lives.

The use of a two-dimensional scale of the Rosser type also rests upon the two untenable assumptions that:
— changes in medical condition are solely a consequence of medical treatment; and
— treatment is the sole function of the health services.

The relationship between patients and the health services

The impact of health services on health remains uncertain. It has been suggested that as many as 80% of people who seek medical attention are neither helped nor harmed in clinical terms, while 10% receive some benefit and an equal number are made worse.[16] One of the major services performed by medical practitioners is reassurance and the alleviation of worry rather than symptoms, most of which disappear of their own accord.

It is also an important function of health service personnel to provide information, advice and help with the making of decisions about matters related to health.[17] Prevention and health promotion featured prominently in the recent consultative document, *The health of the nation*.[18] Welfare, maintenance and care are also major responsibilities of the health services, implying the need to assess process as well as outcome. There may be a great deal of utility in the dynamics and the effects of the system itself.

Mooney has pointed out the danger that QALYs will reinforce the idea that health services are solely about changes in health status related to treatment.[19] If there is more to the NHS than attempting to bring about changes in distress and disability/dependency, there is clearly a need for measures other than QALYs.

The need for patient-orientated measures

If the need for other measures is accepted, it is necessary to be clear about the characteristics of such measures. A great deal of research has been carried out into utilisation of health services, compliance with medical regimens, recovery from illness and judgements of treatment outcome, an overwhelming proportion of which indicates that the perceptions of the patient have a major influence on all these parameters. Thus, while traditionally members of the medical profession have determined the use of resources by deciding when to treat, by which means and where, it is patients who decide whether or not to seek treatment, whether to comply with that treatment, and whether or not to pursue further means of getting the kind of attention that they feel they need. Thus, measures of process and outcome in the health services should be based, wherever feasible, upon the experience, perceptions and preferences of consumers and potential consumers of resources.

From the standpoints of planning, allocation of resources and setting priorities, there are a number of stages in the 'career' of a patient, which makes the judgement of the patient or potential patient of paramount importance.

Utilisation of services

It has long been known that the decision to seek medical attention is more closely linked to how people feel than to their clinical condition.[20] Perceived vulnerability, and an evaluation of the personal, social, occupational and financial costs of being ill play a major role.[21]

For example, there are many more people in the community with symptoms of mental illness than people seeking attention for such symptoms.[22] This may be partly explained by lack of availability and access, but a significant proportion of individuals will not have sought treatment because they feel it is not appropriate or that they would not benefit from it.

Diagnosis

Approximately 50% of the people who *do* seek medical help do not fall into any extant classification of illness, and may be regarded by the doctor as malingering, worried well or hypochondriacal. The patient will most often be told there is 'nothing wrong', or that the doctor cannot find anything wrong. This will be sufficient to reassure some people, but a significant number will continue to feel ill and seek further attention.

Preferences

Studies comparing doctors' assessments of patients' preferences with those of the patients themselves have generally found discrepancies. For example, in an investigation comparing either sparing or amputating a limb in patients with osteosarcoma, the doctors concerned were overwhelmingly of the opinion that patients whose limbs were spared would have a better 'quality of life' than amputees. Subsequent evaluation, using standard measures of social and psychological functioning and the impact of treatment on daily activities, found that the amputees made the better adjustment.[23] Studies of patients with terminal illness have found that up to 90% express a preference for knowing they are dying, whereas up to 90% of doctors think patients would prefer not to know. This finding may reflect more the doctors' reluctance to acknowledge the possibility of death than that of the patients.[24–26]

Compliance

Non-compliance with medical treatment and advice is substantial.[27,28] This is expressed in the form of withdrawal from treatment, failure to adhere to the medical regimen, and not taking prescribed drugs. Studies of prescribing have shown that whereas only 2–5% of patients fail to have their prescriptions made up, between 20 and 80% either do not take the medication or fail to complete the course of treatment.[29]

This imposes unnecessary costs on the NHS, and led Weinstein and Stason to conclude, in relation to hypertensive therapy, that resources would be better invested in improving the compliance of known hypertensive patients than in trying to detect more by screening.[30] However, while much of the literature has been devoted to means of raising compliance levels,[31] many authors acknowledge that non-compliance may be reasonable from the patient's perspective, in terms of unacceptable treatment, inconvenient side-effects, perceived ineffectiveness or unfulfilled expectations.[32,33]

Outcome

Several studies covering a wide range of conditions show discrepancies between doctors and patients in relation to the judged efficacy of treatment. An investigation in Sweden found only 50% agreement between physicians and patients on whether or not treatment had been beneficial.[34] A study of low back pain found even less agreement between the two groups.[35] Similar results have been found in surgery for peptic ulcer,[36] and also in treatment for mental illness.[37] The work of Jachuck *et al.*, which compared the opinions of patients and their relatives with those of the treating physicians about whether or not the patients had improved, found 50% disagreement between doctors and patients and 100% disagreement between relatives and doctors.[38] Clearly, each of the groups concerned use different criteria for their judgements, with doctors focusing on clinical signs and symptoms, and patients being more influenced by how they feel and their ability to fulfil their own expectations. In contrast, relatives are concerned with the demeanour and behaviour of the person with whom they live. However, it is the patient's feelings, supplemented perhaps by the urging of relatives, which influence any further tendency to seek medical attention.

All these factors point to the conclusion that the perceptions of the patient are crucial in determining both the use and the impact of health and medical services. In the past, there has been an unwillingness to give credence to the patient, partly because of a tendency to think of individual patients as misguided at best and malingering at worst. Moreover, there has been a belief that it is not possible to obtain accurate and reliable measures of patients' perceptions of health because these are too 'subjective'. The success and usefulness of patient-completed measures such as the Sickness Impact Profile[39] and the Nottingham Health Profile (NHP)[40] show clearly that these fears are unjustified. There is a need for measures of 'quality of life' firmly grounded in the needs and experiences of the lay public.

Requirements for patient-orientated measures of quality of life

First, a distinction needs to be made between measures which are self-completed by patients and those which reflect the concerns of the patient. The former may be no more than a system which forces the patient to express him or herself in the language and classifications of the health professional or the economist. Measures intended to represent the point of view of the patient must be grounded firmly in material elicited from patients and potential patients. A number of issues must be addressed:

1. Such measures must have a clear conceptual basis which ties them theoretically to changes in quality of life. Currently, the relationship to quality of life is assumed rather than described.
2. The content must apply to all potential respondents, regardless of age, sex, employment and marital status, or socio-economic circumstances. There is a dynamic cognitive and behavioural conflict between the limitations imposed by circumstances (whether from disease or social conditions) and personal needs. This conflict is most often resolved by the latter being tailored to the former.
3. The measurements must be valid, reliable and sensitive to change.
4. The content must be acceptable to respondents, easy to understand and complete. Research has shown that it is possible to involve even those with severe learning disabilities and the mentally ill in the process of evaluation.[41,42]
5. The measures must allow for adaptation to chronic conditions.
6. The measures must be suitable for use in relatively undramatic situations where change is slow, for example, in rehabilitation after an accident.

We have recently attempted to encompass these criteria with the development of a measure of quality of life in depressed patients.[43] This measure was constructed on the basis that quality of life derives from the ability to fulfil human needs, and that many of the activities in which we indulge such as work, social life and hobbies have the latent function of satisfying these needs. Thus, people who are not employed may find alternative means of fulfilling the latent functions of employment. Similarly, individuals whose social and leisure activities are curtailed by illness may find other ways of gaining stimulation, companionship and interest from life. Using models rooted in psychological and sociological theory, a list of needs was drawn up which included needs for affection, self esteem, interest and so on. Interviews were carried out with patients, and the transcripts analysed for suitable questionnaire items which represented aspects of these needs. Drafts of the questionnaire were presented to patients and ex-patients for comment, and field tests were carried out until the content was believed to be acceptable to, and well understood by, lay people. This was followed by more formal tests of validity and reliability, and resulted in a questionnaire which is liked by patients and suitable for use in a wide range of situations — from assessing the efficacy of treatment to judging quality of care and the impact of community care. Above all, the new measure is grounded in a clear conceptual model of quality of life.[43]

Conclusion

A serious problem with current methods for evaluating quality of life is the use of instruments which are neither appropriate nor useful for their intended purpose. Moreover, the criteria for a 'good' measure are often ill understood by the users. Measures that become popular, for example the NHP, are often applied in situations for which they were never intended. In addition, questionnaires 'age' as popular use of language changes and expectations grow. It cannot be taken for granted that a measure which had face validity 15 years ago will retain it today. There is an urgent need for well thought out and theoretically grounded measures in a number of areas which transcend the limitations of QALYs.

More sensitive measures are needed for the assessment of change in conditions which, although not particularly serious, may be very costly because of their widespread nature. For example, there are many competing drug therapies targeted at conditions such as indigestion, influenza, minor skin complaints and so on.

Instruments for the assessment of the quality of life of mentally ill patients and the impact of their care and treatment are also lacking. Although there are several patient-completed questionnaires, they focus on matters of concern to the psychiatrist rather than to the patient. Given that one person in four at some time seeks medical help for a mental problem, and that a large number of alternative psycho-active drugs are now available, this is particularly serious.

Sound measures of patient satisfaction still remain to be developed, which must take into account the understandable tendency of patients to be grateful and relieved after treatment.

Certain groups in society have been almost entirely neglected in relation to quality of life measurement, including:
— ethnic minorities, where cultural differences in perceptions, expectations and language play a significant role in outcome;
— those people who by virtue of mental or physical handicap or illiteracy find it hard to fill in questionnaires, and whose perceptions and requirements may be very different from those of other patients;
— seriously ill and bedridden patients, who are unlikely to improve

very much in terms of disability and dependency but whose quality of life may be significantly influenced by care and management.

Problems peculiar to women have also received little attention in terms of their effect on quality of life and the impact of treatment, yet conditions associated with menstruation, gynaecological problems, pregnancy and the menopause take up a significant proportion of NHS resources. The quality of life of children and infants is another neglected area, and there is a need to explore ways of assessing this, either by developing child-friendly methods or by using patients and carers as proxies.

It would be useful to have techniques for assessing overall quality of life in patients who have recurring acute episodes, for example, those with epilepsy or migraine.

Finally, measures sensitive to non-medical intervention, such as health promotion strategies, prevention, advice and information should be developed.

The current situation in the health service is that inappropriate measures, developed for different purposes, are being forced to do service in situations for which they were never intended and in which they have not been thoroughly tested. It is time for a new set of tools to be devised designed specifically for the tasks in hand. New, improved, valid and reliable measurement is necessary if QALYs are to be used in making decisions about resources. However, there remains an urgent need for a full range of other measures which can be applied to a wider range of patients, in a more comprehensive set of circumstances, and which will allow the expression of views from the consumers of health care services.

References

1. Walsh R, Aranha G, Freeark R. Mortality and quality of life after total abdominal colectomy. *Archives of Surgery.* 1990; **125**: 1564–6
2. Croog S, Levine S, Testa M, Brown B. The effects of anti-hypertensive therapy on quality of life. *New England Journal of Medicine* 1986; **314**: 1657–64
3. Williams A. The economics of coronary by-pass grafting. *British Medical Journal* 1985; **291**: 326–9
4. Parsons T. *The social system.* New York: Free Press, 1952
5. Kelman S. The social nature of the definition problem in health. *International Journal of Health Services* 1975; **5**: 625–42
6. Rosser R, Kind P. A scale for valuations of states of illness: is there a consensus? *International Journal of Epidemiology* 1978; **7**: 347–57
7. Rosser R, Watts V. The measurement of hospital output. *International Journal of Epidemiology* 1972; **1**: 361–8

8. Carr-Hill R. Background material for the workshop on QALYs: assumptions of the QALY procedure. *Social Science and Medicine* 1989; **29**: 469–77

9. Carr-Hill R. Current practice in obtaining the 'Q' in QALYs: a cautionary note. *British Medical Journal* 1991; **303**: 699–701

10. Carr-Hill R. Allocating resources to health care: is the QALY (quality-adjusted life year) a technical solution to a political problem? *International Journal of Health Services* 1991; **21**: 351–63

11. Rawles J. Castigating QALYs. *Journal of Medical Ethics* 1989; **15**: 143–7

12. Gudex C, Kind P. The QALY toolkit. *Discussion Paper No. 38*. York: Centre for Health Economics, Health Economics Consortium, 1988

13. Euroqol Group. Euroqol—a new facility for the measurement of health-related quality of life. *Health Policy* 1990; **16**: 199–208

14. McKenna S, Hunt S. *An assessment of measures available for evaluating the treatment of intractable epilepsy*. Manchester: Galen Research and Consultancy Research Report, 1990

15. World Health Organisation. *International classification of impairments, disabilities and handicaps*. Geneva: WHO, 1980

16. McKeown T. *The role of medicine: dream, mirage or nemesis*. Oxford: Basil Blackwell, 1984

17. Strull W, Lo B, Charles G. Do patients want to participate in medical decision making? *Journal of the American Medical Association* 1984; **252**: 2990–4

18. Department of Health. *The health of the nation: a consultative document for health in England*. London: HMSO, 1991

19. Mooney G. QALYs: are they enough? A health economist's perspective. *Journal of Medical Ethics* 1989; **15**: 148–52

20. Anderson J, Buck C, Danaher K, Fry J. Users and non-users of doctors: implications for self care. *Journal of the Royal College of General Practitioners* 1977; **27**: 155–9

21. Becker M, ed. The health belief model and personal health behaviour. *Health Education Monographs* 1974; **2**: 324–508

22. Goldberg D, Huxley P. *Mental illness in the community: the pathway to psychiatric care*. London: Tavistock, 1980

23. Sugarbaker P, Barofsky I, Rosenberg S, Gianola F. Quality of life assessment of patients in extremity sarcoma clinical trials. *Surgery* 1982; **91**: 17–23

24. Feiffel H. Death. In: Farberow N, ed. *Taboo topics*. London: Prentice Hall, 1963

25. Crane D. Dying and its dilemmas: a field of research. In: Brim O, Freeman H, Levine S, Scotch N, eds. *The dying patient*. New York: Russell Sage Foundation, 1970

26. Lasagna L. Physicians' behaviour towards the dying patient. In: Brim O, Freeman H, Levine S, Scotch N, eds. *The dying patient*. New York: Russell Sage Foundation, 1970

27. Mitchell J. Compliance with medical regimens: an annotated bibliography. *Health Education Monographs* 1974; **2**: 75

28. Stimson G. Obeying doctor's orders: a view from the other side. *Social Science and Medicine* 1974; **8**: 97–104

29. Cartwright A. *Health surveys in practice and potential*. London: King Edward's Hospital Fund for London, 1983

30. Weinstein M, Stason W. Foundations of cost-effectiveness analysis for health and medical practices. *New England Journal of Medicine* 1977; **296**: 716–21
31. Ley P. Psychological studies of doctor-patient communication. In: Rachman S, ed. *Contributions to medical psychology*. Oxford and New York: Pergamon Press, 1977
32. Becker M, Maiman L. Models of health-related behaviour. In: Mechanic D, ed. *Handbook of health, health care and the health professions*. New York: The Free Press, 1983: 539–68
33. Conrad P. The meaning of medications: another look at compliance. *Social Science and Medicine* 1985; **20**: 29–37
34. Orth-Gomer K, Britton M, Rehnqvist N. Quality of care in an outpatient department: the patients' view. *Social Science and Medicine* 1979; **13A**: 347–51
35. Thomas M, Lyttle D. Patient expectations about success of treatment and reported relief from low back pain. *Journal of Psychosomatic Research* 1980; **24**: 297–301
36. Hall R, Horrocks J, Clamp S, DeDombal F. Observer variation in assessment of results of surgery for peptic ulceration. *British Medical Journal* 1976; **274**: 814–6
37. Prusoff B, Klerman G, Paykel E. Concordance between clinical assessments and patients' self report in depression. *Archives of General Psychiatry* 1972; **26**: 546–52
38. Jachuck S, Brierley H, Jachuck S, Willcox P. The effect of hypotensive drugs on quality of life. *Journal of the Royal College of General Practitioners* 1982; **32**: 103–5
39. Bergner M, Bobbitt R, Pollard W, Martin D, Gilson B. The Sickness Impact Profile: development and final revision of a health status measure. *Medical Care* 1976; **19**: 787–805
40. Hunt S, McEwen J, McKenna S. *Measuring health status*. London: Croom Helm, 1986
41. Stanley B, Roy A. Evaluating the quality of life of people with mental handicap. *Mental Health Review* 1988; **1**: 197–210
42. Lehman A, Ward N, Linn L. Chronic mental patients: the quality of life issue. *American Journal of Psychiatry* 1982; **139**: 1271–5
43. Hunt S, McKenna S. The LQD: a scale for the measurement of quality of life in depression. *Social Science and Medicine* (submitted)

DISCUSSION

Azim Lakhani: The thrust of the chapter largely rejects professional judgement, but recommends that of the patient or the public. The answer must surely be a balance of the two tailored to the circumstances. Most people recognise some of the inadequacies of professional judgement, but there is room for both this and patient perspectives. In the treatment of asymptomatic disease or modification of a pathology, professional judgement may have a significant role to play.

I was interested in the authors' arguments about the way people adapt, particularly to chronic conditions, which raises the issues of under-valuation, whose valuation are we talking about and in what circumstances are those valuations obtained. Is it the public's valuations, asking people to imagine a certain state and place a value on it, or the valuations of people who have experienced the particular condition? Other things to take into account are whether the valuations are made by people who have knowledge that effective interventions are available that would make life more tolerable, a knowledge influenced by having relatives or friends who suffered from a condition who may have expressed views in certain ways, and so on.

Clive Smee: Whose valuation is to be taken into account, linked to the purpose for which these valuations are to be used, seems to be critical. I suspect that we all think of this in terms of the decisions in which we or those with whom we work may be involved—which are often very different kinds of decisions. When I am in an aeroplane flying through an area of turbulence I wonder why the airline has not supplied all passengers with parachutes, but when I buy a ticket I am glad it did not, and that the ticket is cheap. I use this metaphor to illustrate that anybody who has an illness, particularly one seen as life-threatening, may feel that all conceivable resources should be put into that illness, but tougher decisions have to be made at some level in government unless the need for rationing of health resources is not accepted.

Nick Ross: There are fundamentally two different sorts of priorities. The first affects the individual clinician faced with an individual patient. The principal theme of this chapter is that 'respect for the patient should be paramount'. I do not believe this makes much sense. When a clinician is faced with the consequences of a serious accident in which 15 people have been hurt, most of them unconscious, he will decide his priorities for action. It is not a matter of telling the first patient that he will now bestow upon him his skills regardless of whether that patient is one of the least injured or is about to die. As has been observed earlier, doctors are not trained to think about resource allocation, but about 'the patient' as an individual. This is a fraud; it produces a sort of innumeracy, a wilful ignorance by the medical profession of the existence of many more dilemmas than the obvious ones with which they have to cope.

The second kind of priority, resource allocation, falls into two separate areas: first, how the government, the NHS, the region, even the unit, describe how resources are allocated on a political scale and, secondly, how the individual doctor allocates his resources within the framework set out by his unit, region or country.

The two types of priority require different judgements. One may respond well to QALYs, which may enable managers to set priorities, but the other, individual, level is not so amenable to QALYs, at least not in their current rather crude state. I think the authors are right to call the technology primitive. Surely the first step is not to give doctors in acute medicine a tool like a QALY and tell them to look up the patient's problem in the table and decide whether or not to operate, or give the drugs. QALYs cannot be a substitute for knowledge. The doctor must have a broader responsibility.

In industry, there is enormous interest at the moment in giving all members of staff, whether junior or senior, some education about 'commerce' — an understanding of the principles of business, so that the metal riveter understands how and why profits are important, and how a company does or does not survive. Employers used to fear that such information would make members of staff better trade unionists, but now there is a recognition that everybody must pull together in order to make an enterprise work. Similarly, before asking doctors to apply QALYs, they should be asked to think more broadly about the resource implications of what they do.

Sonja Hunt: If the term 'quality of life' is used, the patient's view should be primarily taken into account. If priorities are set in some other way, without that term, we must not imply to the public that these decisions are based upon information about how the quality of life of patients will be affected.

Clive Smee: The issue of which kinds of decisions we are talking about is important and underlies a lot of the tension in the field. If we think QALYs are primitive, what about the mechanisms used to arrive at decisions now at higher levels of administration? If a Minister asks any of his officials, whether doctors, economists or administrators, to summarise the benefits that will result from putting £20 million into one programme compared with putting the same sum into another, what are the alternatives to using something like a QALY — what set of indicators can be used?

Henry Neuberger: Azim Lakhani mentioned the relationship between professional judgement and people's perceptions. I think that QALYs should be seen as a way of standing between, on the one hand, what would be universally acknowledged to be professional clinical judgement, which is knowing what happens to people after certain medical interventions and, on the other hand, what would be recognised as individual, personal, lay judgement, which is what people feel about what happens to them when they undergo a medical intervention. We are arguing about defining the space that lies between.

In commenting on Alan Williams' article on coronary artery bypass grafting, Ian Russell (page 49) pointed to what has always been to me a difficulty about this. Alan Williams asked some doctors about outcomes of this intervention but, as Ian Russell said, even the quite large range of outcomes described represented only a very small part of those clinically possible. Clinical trials can make only some probabilistic statements about some impacts of any intervention. On the other hand, economists want answers to all the questions if they are to make any judgements. The people who undergo these interventions do not have much idea of what anybody else is talking about. A means of communication has to be found; economists, psychologists or anyone else can be no more than brokers between professional judgement and lay opinion. If simple measures of quality of life are abandoned, the end result will be asking lay people to make professional clinical judgements. A way of drawing in clinicians should be sought in which they are able to describe outcomes in a way comprehensible to lay people. Also, designers of surveys should try to construct their descriptions in such a way that people can place valuations on them. Once this problem is solved, all the intermediate professionals can withdraw.

Douglas Black: As Nick Ross pointed out, decisions about the individual patient and decisions about the provision of resources have to be considered. Surely an intermediate area also to be considered is definable groups of patients. If I may be dogmatic, I cannot see formal analysis of the quality of life making any contribution to clinicians' decisions on what to do for individual patients, although such an analysis must make a marginal contribution to the general medical and nursing outlook on how to treat specified groups of patients. However, I can see a big future for the application of measures of the quality of life in allocating resources, provided that there is a greater refinement in our ethical understanding.

Peter Selby: The principle of any system of clinical measurement is to choose the method to suit the purpose. For instance, if the purpose is how to allocate resources, a method of measurement that addresses that is needed. This is what Alan Williams is trying to do, and it is generally agreed that there is more work to be done in this field. Similarly, if the purpose is the care of an individual patient, a suitable measure for that purpose is chosen or, if a sophisticated evaluation of the psychosocial well-being of a cancer patient is being undertaken, one of the questionnaires designed for this particular purpose will be used.

The definition of quality of life chosen will vary according to the purpose to which the data will be put. It is reasonable to say '*this* is how I am going to define quality of life in this context, *this* is how I shall try to seek answers as to how to measure it, and *these* are the results'. There is not likely to be one all-embracing, all-purposeful definition of quality of life.

Hopefully, doctors will graduate who are more informed about issues relating to quality and about functional and psychological outcomes. Most of what is being discussed and used now in relation to techniques of measurement and allocation of resources may not be considered useful in five years' time, but the educational spin-off of this area of enquiry will be valuable.

Most of the clinicians with whom I work are concerned about these issues, and about getting good functional and psychological out-comes—although they do not always know how to achieve them, and certainly not how to measure what they do. It is a mistake to believe that clinicians resist these ideas, but there is a measure of anxiety about how they should proceed.

7 | Index of health-related quality of life

Rachel Rosser, Michaela Cottee, Rosalind Rabin and Caroline Selai
Department of Academic Psychiatry, University College & Middlesex School of Medicine, London

Introduction

This chapter outlines the on-going development of an instrument to measure health-related quality of life, the Index of Health-Related Quality of Life (IHQL). The first section describes the current status of the IHQL and includes a brief description of the instrument, together with details of a number of application studies in which the IHQL is currently being employed. Some aspects of the development of the IHQL which we hope to complete shortly will be described. Finally, for the sake of completeness, some of the developmental work which remains to be tackled (subject to the continuation of funds) will be outlined.

The development of any new instrument to measure health-related quality of life is time-consuming and labour-intensive if it is to be conducted scrupulously. We hope to be able to demonstrate that the IHQL is potentially a valid, reliable and useful instrument. Without full reliability and validity testing, however, a note of caution should be sounded about its use.

IHQL: current status

Description of instrument

The IHQL provides a broad and sensitive measure of social, psychological and physical functioning, and is designed to be applicable across all diagnostic groups. It is based on a five-level multidimensional classification system, but it is possible to derive an assessment of health status on a single unidimensional scale. Thus, the IHQL combines the advantages of a global index with those of a profile instrument, and is potentially of use both in clinical research and for informing clinical audit and policy decisions.

81

The first stage in the development of the IHQL was the derivation of a three-dimensional classification system from the original two-dimensional Rosser Index based on the dimensions of disability and distress.[1,2] Distress was separated into physical and emotional components, to give the three dimensions of disability, (physical) discomfort and (emotional) distress. The levels of each of these dimensions are presented in Appendix 1 (page 147).* Valuations for the 175 composite health states which can be described using the three-dimensional classification system (excluding unconsciousness) were obtained using standard gamble for states of one year's duration and are presented in Appendix 2 (page 149).

In developing the IHQL, the three dimensions of disability, discomfort and distress have been subdivided into seven attributes (dependency, dysfunction, pain/discomfort, symptoms, dysphoria, disharmony and fulfilment), which in turn have been further subdivided into 44 scales. There are 107 descriptors which are subsumed by these scales with 225 descriptor levels between them. The resultant hierarchical structure, which makes it possible to use the IHQL both as a global index and a profile instrument, is presented in Appendix 3 (page 150).

The descriptors were derived through a questionnaire survey of a random sample of the population of Bloomsbury Health District, in the course of psychometric interviews with health professionals and others, and from a review of the relevant literature and of other instruments which purport to measure health-related quality of life.[3] Descriptors were eliminated only if they were redundant through duplication. In this way, the final set of descriptors is intended to describe as comprehensively as possible the many ways in which the condition of a person's health may affect his or her quality of life. (Note that the IHQL is concerned entirely with health and not with the wider issue of the effect of social deprivation on quality of life.)

The descriptors have been incorporated into an IHQL questionnaire for use in clinical settings in order to assess health-related quality of life. Three versions of the IHQL questionnaire are being produced.†
— a self-complete version to be completed by the patient;
— an observer-complete version to be completed by a trained observer on behalf of the patient in an interview situation;
— a relative-rated version to be completed on behalf of the patient by a relative or close friend.

---

*Appendices to this chapter are given at the end of the book.

†Copies of the IHQL can be obtained by researchers interested in using the instrument upon application to the authors. Software for data entry is being prepared, and will also be available upon application to the authors.

Derivation of scale values

In order for the IHQL to be used to measure health-related quality of life, it is necessary to attach values to the health states which can be described using the instrument. The number of composite health states which it is theoretically possible to describe using the 107 descriptors is in the order of 10^{52}. Like the number of theoretically possible composite health states, the cognitive complexity of scaling these states would be unimaginably vast. It would be impossible to use an established scaling technique such as standard gamble to obtain scale values for all possible health states, although it may be possible to scale subsets of health state descriptors in this way using an incomplete blocks design. However, this would still be a complex and methodologically unsatisfactory compromise. A novel multistage category-rating technique based on multi-attribute theory[4] has therefore been developed. Torrance *et al.* modified this approach in order to obtain values in two stages.[5] However, we have extended the approach, and have applied it in six stages in order to obtain scale values for use with the IHQL. The six-stage category-rating technique was first described by Allison.[6]

The scaling task requires the use of 101 11-point category rating scales:

Stage 1: the levels of the descriptors are rated relative to the most severe level.

Stage 2: the descriptors are rated relative to each other on the appropriate scales.

Stage 3: the scales are rated relative to each other on the appropriate attributes.

Stage 4: the attributes are rated relative to each other on the appropriate dimensions.

Stage 5: the three dimensions are rated relative to each other.

Stage 6: the worst possible combination of all the descriptors (equivalent to extreme disability with extreme discomfort and extreme distress) are rated relative to being dead on a single scale.

At the first stage in the derivation of the scale values, the rating for the worst possible combination of the descriptors is scaled relative to being dead. This will result in a 0–1 scale of values with 1 corresponding to being dead, and 0 corresponding to no impairment. At the second stage, the ratings for each of the dimensions are re-scaled relative to the worst possible state. The attributes are then re-scaled relative to the dimensions, the scales relative to the attributes, and the most extreme levels of the descriptors re-scaled relative to the scales. At the sixth and final stage, the levels of the descriptors themselves are re-scaled. The final values obtained correspond to the disutilities of the levels of each descriptor.

It is possible to derive values for any combination of the health state descriptors. Thus, it is possible to make an assessment of the effect of any condition upon health-related quality of life, and so make cross-diagnostic comparisons. By summing all the applicable disutilities and subtracting the total from 1, a single value for health-related quality of life is derived on the usual 0–1 death-health scale, where 1 corresponds to no impairment in health-related quality of life and 0 to states equivalent to death. Negative values correspond to states worse than death. Positive health attributes (eg a 'fighting' attitude to illness) may offset these negative values. It is also possible to aggregate or dis-aggregate the values over the five levels in order to derive profiles of values. Because of the comprehensiveness of the descriptive system and the different levels of aggregation, the IHQL allows greater descriptive detail than do other instruments, and it is hoped that it will show greater sensitivity to clinical changes.

Provisional scale values have been obtained using a convenience sample of 40 subjects and are also in Appendix 3.

Reliability and validity testing

In developing a new instrument to measure health-related quality of life, it is essential to make a thorough assessment of the reliability and validity of the instrument. In other words, does the instrument measure what it claims to measure (validity), and how consistently does it measure what it measures (reliability)? Given the novelty of the scaling technique to obtain the scale values used in conjunction with the IHQL questionnaires, the properties of the multistage category-rating technique have to be assessed as well as those of the questionnaires themselves.

Multistage category-rating technique No assessment has yet been made of the test-retest reliability of the scaling method, the stability of the ratings obtained over time, the consensus of the values obtained from different sample groups, or the comparability of the values obtained using multistage category-rating with those obtained using other, established scaling techniques. However, values obtained by applying multistage category-rating in three stages to the original three-dimensional classification system have been shown to have a power relationship with values obtained using standard gamble. Some assessment has also been made of the degree of agreement between the raters in the convenience sample by examination of the variance of the ratings made.

IHQL questionnaires It is necessary to make some assessment of reliability and validity for each of the three different versions of the IHQL. Test-retest reliability has not yet been assessed adequately for any version of the IHQL.

In a pilot study involving 4 raters and 12 patients, the inter-rater reliability of the observer-complete version was high. No assessment has yet been made of the inter-rater reliability of the relative-rated version. It is not appropriate to assess inter-rater reliability for the self-complete version.

In the absence of any gold standard criterion by which instruments which purport to measure health-related quality of life can be validated, it is necessary to investigate the convergent validity of the IHQL with other instruments. The overall IHQL score has been shown to correlate highly with the total score on the General Health Questionnaire (GHQ)[7] and the Symptom Checklist (SCL-90),[8] but not so well with the Impact of Events Scale (IES).[9] It should soon be possible to make some assessment of the convergent validity of the IHQL in relation to the Brief Psychiatric Rating Scale (BPRS) for psychiatric patients. No comparisons with other measures of health-related quality of life have been made at this stage, although studies are planned.

Application studies using the IHQL

The Daily Living Programme study is designed to compare treatment on this programme with orthodox inpatient treatment for psychiatric patients at the Maudsley Hospital in an analysis of cost-utility.[10] The observer-complete version of the IHQL was employed. Preliminary analysis of the time 1 (admission) and time 2 (three months after admission) data for the 59 patients in each group who have so far been tested on both occasions shows that, on the whole, both forms of treatment lead to a significant improvement in health-related quality of life, but analysis at the more detailed levels of the IHQL reveals some interesting differences between the two patient groups. A more complete analysis is planned to involve observations of the entire sample (175) at four time points over an 18-month period which may yield a more detailed profile of outcomes in this unique study.

The IHQL is being employed by the Stress Clinic at the Middlesex Hospital in a randomised controlled trial to assess the effect of a waiting list period prior to psychotherapy upon the health-related quality of life of disaster victims. This study also permits comparisons between the

IHQL and a range of psychiatric and social measures, which should be indicative of the convergent validity of the IHQL.

The IHQL is also being used in a long-term study of a psychosomatic ward associated with University College and Middlesex School of Medicine. For the past $2^{1}/_{2}$ years, patients have been assessed at admission and discharge using the self-complete version of the IHQL, the observer-complete version, and the BPRS. During this time, the ward has been relocated three times with associated changes in operational policy. This study therefore provides a unique opportunity to monitor many aspects of the health-related quality of life of the patients on the ward over a long time period.

Time factors

Studies by Butler and Rosser indicate the following time-related factors:[11,12]

1. The utility assigned to states of varying duration is *not* independent of the variable being measured; eg disability diminishes in importance over time, whereas pain increases.
2. Over very long time periods (50 years) health-related quality of life is discounted. Over shorter periods (10 years) no discounting occurs. This effect may have increased over the past 15 years, and is consistent with changes in the impact of educational policies concerned with forgoing present pleasures to minimise the risks to future health.

IHQL: on-going work

Scaling study

A large scaling study is under way, which will enable an assessment to be made of the consensus between different groups of subjects (patients, doctors, nurses and the general public), and which will result in definitive scale values for use with the IHQL. It will also be possible to investigate the relationship between ratings, some of which appear to be positive, and various features of the subjects such as age, sex, occupation, education, religion, ethnic origin, personality, and experience of illness in self and others.

The consent of consultants in orthopaedics, neurology, oncology and surgery has already been obtained, and 100 patients are to be recruited across these specialties. Over 100 members of the general public have also been recruited in a two-stage random selection process. We hope to follow up some of the subjects in order to assess the test-retest reliability and stability of the ratings obtained.

Interview probe

A small-scale study has started which will probe in more detail the responses made on the self-complete version of the IHQL, in order to compare a patient's verbal account of his or her health state with the responses made on the IHQL questionnaire. Discrepancies may be a feature of the amount of insight that patients have into their condition, of their ease of comprehension and completion of the questionnaire, or differences in the use of language and underlying concepts.

Application studies

Further analysis of the data collected from the Daily Living Programme is planned (see earlier section), including more detailed analysis of the time 1 and time 2 data, preliminary analysis of the time 3 (nine months after admission) and, hopefully, analysis of the longer-term changes. This will constitute a unique cost-utility analysis of a mental health programme. Further analysis of the data from the psychotherapy trial on disaster victims is also planned, including assessment of the significance of changes over time.

Initial analysis of the data being collected from the psychosomatic ward has been carried out (to be published). Data collection is ongoing.

IHQL: future work

1. Analysis of the data from the IHQL scaling study and interpretation of the results.
2. Extension of the scaling study to assess test-retest reliability and stability so far as is possible.
3. Assessment of the test-retest reliability of the three versions of the IHQL.
4. Further assessment of the convergent validity of the IHQL, together with its sensitivity and specificity. For example, no comparison has yet been made using other established instruments which are used to measure health-related quality of life, such as the Nottingham Health Profile (NHP) or the Sickness Impact Profile (SIP).
5. Further assessment of the inter-rater reliability of the observer-complete version, and assessment of the inter-rater reliability of the relative-rated version.
6. Comparison of the three versions of the IHQL, in terms both of their reliability and validity, and of the equivalence of the

results obtained by applying the different instruments to the same patients.

7. Further assessment of the validity of the descriptors, with the possibility of producing a shorter version of the IHQL. It is also hoped to produce versions for people with special problems connected with homelessness, overcrowding or minority status.

8. Validation of the hierarchical structure and the testing of the impact of the structure imposed upon the scale values obtained.

9. Comparison of the IHQL with the three-dimensional classification system in utility terms (assessments on the three-dimensional classification system are being made alongside the administration of the IHQL questionnaires).

10. Comparison of multistage category-rating with other, established methods of scaling.

11. Consideration of the incorporation of individual valuations.

12. The continued development of a data-handling programme which assists in the inputting of patients' responses on to computer in a form suitable for use with statistical packages. This programme could be extended to handle the aggregation of the scale values, thus opening up the possibility of simultaneous data collection and assessment of quality of life using a PC or lap-top computer.

13. Further consideration of the technical, ethical and philosophical assumptions connected with quality of life measurement, together with some assessment of their pertinence to the IHQL.

At a more practical level, the production of a unique data entry and analysis software package is envisaged within the next year.

Acknowledgements

The principal author thanks the Department of Health for funding during 1969–91. We also thank Carole Butler and Richard Allison for scaling work, and our scaling subjects for their industry and patience.

References

1. Rosser RM, Watts VC. The measurement of hospital output. *International Journal of Epidemiology* 1972; **1**: 361–8

2. Rosser RM, Watts VC. The measurement of illness. *Journal of the Operational Research Society* 1978; **29**: 529–40

3. Butler C, Rabin R, Rosser R. Health-related quality of life: a study of descriptors elicited from a random sample of Bloomsbury District residents (in preparation)

4. Keeney RL, Raiffa H. *Decisions with multiple objectives: preferences and value trade-offs*. New York: Wiley, 1976

5. Torrance GW, Boyle MH, Horwood SP. Application of multi-attribute utility theory to measure social preferences for health states. *Operations Research* 1982; **30**: 1043–69

6. Allison R. Presentation at the Priory Fellows Research Symposium (8 February 1990)

7. Goldberg DP, Hillies VF. A scaled version of the General Health Questionnaire. *Psychological Medicine* 1979; **9**: 139–45

8. Derogatis LR. *SCL–90–R: administration scoring and procedures manual.* I. Baltimore: Clinical Psychometric Research, 1977

9. Horowitz M, Wilner N, Alvarez W. Impact of Events Scale: a measure of subjective stress. *Psychosomatic Medicine* 1979; **41**(3): 209–18

10. Marks I, Connolly J, Muijen M. The Maudsley Daily Living Programme. A controlled cost-effectiveness study of community-based versus standard in-patient care of serious mental illness. *Bulletin of the Royal College of Psychiatrists* 1988; **11**: 22–3

11. Butler C, Rosser R. Health-related quality of life: valuation of states of different durations using standard gamble (in preparation)

12. Butler C, Rosser R. Time factors in health state utility measurement: the valuation of illness at different times in the future (in preparation)

DISCUSSION

Roy Carr-Hill: Some sort of Ptolemaic complexity seems to be emerging, and perhaps a Galileo is needed to tell us how to start again. The people asked to do the valuations in this study seem to have had to make 386 separate valuations (although I presume some sampling or choice may be possible). At any rate, this is my impression from the staged way in which the valuations are made. Paul Kind and colleagues reported that one of their problems with the valuations by time trade off and standard gamble was that people were asked to make so many valuations—although, in fact, the number was only a handful compared to 386. Because of this, each respondent was actually asked to make only a small number of valuations, which was thought partly to explain the inconsistency in the results (Table 5, page 29).

Yet a lay person would say that Rachel Rosser's scheme is *still* not comprehensive because it does not take into account the extent to which the patient feels in control and can respond to what is happening. This is not included in the IHQL—or in any other health-related quality of life measure.

Rachel Rosser has presented work in progress, so understandably cannot say much about specific results. I look forward to seeing the evidence that there is a power relationship between the multistage category-rating and the values obtained by the standard gamble technique.

Rachel Rosser: Despite the extent of detail, it is correct to say that the IHQL is still not comprehensive. Obviously, some of the descriptors will be essentially redundant, in that they may not contribute much to the overall score. Our research team includes a philosopher, a neuro-psychologist and sociologists, who are all trying to discover the mental model of the individual respondent. We have tried to follow this in increasing depth since first publishing on this topic in 1972.

Michaela Cottee: The scaling task has been made as simple as possible, and we believe it is still a valid approach. Category rating was chosen in the hope that this is a more intuitive task for the respondent than something like standard gamble which contains all sorts of gambling concepts. Respondents also rate the individual levels of the descriptors as opposed to composite states. To scale huge numbers of composite states using a technique like standard gamble is a complex task. In the intermediate stage in the development of the IHQL, Rachel Rosser's original two-dimensional classification was divided into a three-dimensional classification, and some work was done comparing standard gamble and composite states and a multistage category-rating approach, which lends some validity to the approach. This is when the power relationship was found which agrees with the power relationship found for the two techniques by Torrance.[1]

Reference

1. Torrance GW. Social preferences for health states: an empirical evaluation of three measurement techniques. *Socioeconomic Planning Sciences* 1976; **10**: 129–36

8 | Measurement of the quality of life: the particular problems of cancer patients

Peter Selby

Director, Institute for Cancer Studies, St James's University Hospital, Leeds

Introduction

Issues relating to the measurement of quality of life have a special importance in the practice of cancer medicine. The problems of cancer patients, whether physical, psychological or social, are well recognised and well documented. However, the practice of cancer medicine differs in a number of ways, some of them qualitatively, from the treatment of other common diseases. These differences generate particular problems both in the measurement of quality of life and in the development of appropriate measurement methods. I will argue that decision taking in clinical oncology is achieved by balancing the limited efficacy of treatments against their probable or possible toxicities, and that this balance must take into account the patients' wishes. Patients need to know the likely impact of any treatment on the quality of their lives overall (the net outcome of efficacy and toxicity). Measurement of quality of life is therefore particularly desirable — as well as being rather difficult.

There has been over a decade of work towards the development of methods for measuring quality of life in cancer patients, but a satisfactory instrument for all purposes, fulfilling all recognised requirements, has yet to be devised. In a recent review of available instruments, a working party of the Medical Research Council (MRC) Cancer Therapy Committee concluded that:

> a multidimensional scale which is specific to patients with cancer, meets all the assessment criteria and provides scores which have relevance to clinical judgements remains to be developed.[1]

Limitations on instruments include the scope of enquiry, design and interpretation. Only a limited number of instruments have been subjected to rigorous psychometric evaluation for reliability, validity and structure.[2-10]

This chapter will discuss four main issues:

1. The main factors which determine quality of life in cancer patients, with particular reference to breast cancer.
2. The special difficulties in measuring quality of life in cancer patients.
3. The available methods of measurement.
4. Possible approaches to the measurement of quality of life, and a proposal for a simple pragmatic approach, drawing on defined factors, and describing a substantial part of quality of life in most people.

Factors which determine quality of life in cancer patients

In 1984, we reported the development of a method for assessing the quality of life of breast cancer patients based on self-assessment by multiple linear analogue scales.[11] The questionnaire contained 31 items assessed by patients' self-report, including 18 about general health problems derived from the Sickness Impact Profile (SIP)[12] and 13 about major problems associated with breast cancer. The method is designed to allow exchange of the items related to breast cancer for those related to other cancer sites. The reliability and validity of the measurement method in the original study, carried out in Toronto, Canada, was reported. The questionnaire performed well in reliability and validity studies, and achieved standards which were felt to be acceptable for an instrument used in a research setting.[11]

In evaluation of the performance of a questionnaire of this kind, an important test is the examination of the correlations between individual questions. The techniques of factor analysis[13] are used to deduce common factors to which the individual items are correlated, and the results of such analysis are known as the factor structure of the data. In the data collected in the Canadian study (96 patients), a five-factor structure was obtained from the questionnaire. Factors were identified relating to activities of everyday living, symptoms, emotional well-being, alimentary well-being and appearance/attractiveness. These factors represent the main features of quality of life when assessed in this way. Results from further work in the UK using the factor analysis approach in a larger patient group (294)[14] (Table 1) show a close relationship to the Canadian results in that the factors derived include activities of daily living, emotional well-being and alimentary symptoms. The other items are not associated so closely into distinct factors. The extensive work required to explore the analysis fully is

Table 1. Correlation between items: results of factor analysis. All patients, all 28 items.[14]

Item	Factor				
	1	2	3	4	5
Housework	0.76				
Mobility around home, town, country	0.72				
Regular out of home employment	0.67				
Physical activity		0.66			
Social life outside the family	0.65				
Recreation pastimes or hobbies	0.63				
Fatigue	0.62				
Sexual activity	0.62				
Eating disturbance	0.60				
Bowel disturbance	0.58				
Pain	0.51				
Sleeping disturbance	0.50	(0.46)			
Attractiveness to the opposite sex	0.43				
Depression		0.73			
Level of anxiety			0.69		
Appearance of your body		0.68			
Anger		0.68			
Family relationships		0.64			
Speech				0.72	
Writing			0.61		
Breathing			0.60		
Information		(0.40)	0.55		
Concentration		(0.49)	0.50		
Vomiting				0.87	
Nausea					0.84
Sore mouth				0.52	
Self-care (washing, dressing)					0.67
Hair loss					0.55

Figures shown are rotated factor loadings. Figures in parentheses indicate secondary factor loadings >0.4.

beyond the scope of this chapter, but is published elsewhere.[14] However, the results are reassuringly consistent internally, and also with other studies using quite different approaches.

It is not thought that further factor analyses will define more precisely the factors that determine quality of life in our cancer patients. For instance, our results are broadly in agreement with the studies carried out using the Rotterdam Symptom Checklist.[15] In that questionnaire, both psychological and physical distress together with alimentary features are separate factors in two of the three factor analyses, but alimentary symptoms are difficult to analyse in the third study because of skewed distribution of answers. Schipper *et al.* identified physical well-being, emotional state and nausea as distinct factors but, in addition, their questionnaire considered aspects of family hardship and disruption which emerged as a separate factor.[16]

The special difficulties measuring quality of life in cancer patients

Difficulties related to disease

The physical dimension The symptoms associated with local or advanced cancer are many and varied. The prognosis of the cancer patient will depend greatly upon the site of his primary cancer and the stage of disease, but for many common cancers the long-term prognosis is still extremely poor. Although the severity of symptoms and the threat to patients' lives for many cancers may not be greater than for other common life-threatening conditions such as ischaemic heart disease, they present special difficulties in the measurement of quality of life arising from the multiplicity of cancer presentations and disabilities. Each cancer site is associated with a spectrum of presentations and stages, and the measurement of quality of life needs to encompass all of these. This presents a problem in the generation of generic instruments, which has yet to be adequately addressed. In an attempt to address this, we proposed the possibility of creating modular questionnaires with a core of generic questions and a range of optional questions relating to different cancer sites. This approach has some attractions. The model, developed for generic application and for application to breast cancer, is shown in Table 2 (which also indicates reliability for the items).[11]

In addition to the problems presented by the multiplicity of cancer presentations, their severity can generate restrictions on the measurement of quality of life. The ill patient with advanced and/or recurrent cancer requires extensive and intensive care, and it is important that the measurement of quality of life in this context be not onerous for the patient. The reduction of questionnaires to the minimum possible is necessary, but this compounds the difficulties presented by the many features that must be measured.

Psychological problems Cancer patients suffer depression and anxiety and frequently experience anger as a reaction to their illness. They are,

Table 2. Test-retest reliability of items in a linear analogue self-assessment quality of life questionnaire.[11]

Item	r	Item	r
General health item			
Work	1.00	Recreation	0.78
Increased eating	0.96	Social life	0.75
Writing	0.92	Housework	0.74
Anger	0.90	Reduced eating	0.72
Reduced sleep	0.82	Physical activity	0.70
Concentration	0.81	Family relations	0.70
Self-care	0.81	Anxiety	0.64
Depression	0.80	Mobility	0.63
Increased sleep	0.79	Speech	0.78
Disease-related item			
Dysuria	0.85	Sore mouth	0.68
Attractiveness	0.84	Breathing	0.66
Pain	0.83	Fatigue	0.66
Information	0.79	Diarrhoea	0.37
Constipation	0.79	Nausea	0.32
Hair loss	0.78	Vomiting	0.25
Appearance	0.78	Uniscale[22]	0.72

Correlation coefficients (r) are highly significant: $p < 0.001$, except those for diarrhoea ($p = 0.005$), nausea ($p = 0.002$) and vomiting ($p = 0.012$).

of course, not alone in experiencing emotional disorder as a result of the presence of physical illness but, again, there are particular aspects of their illness which makes the measurement of quality of life in this context especially difficult. Emotional well-being is an independent factor determining quality of life for cancer patients which requires measurement (Table 1).

One reason why the screening of cancer patients for psychiatric morbidity by psychometric questionnaires is more difficult than for other diseases is technical and relates to the construction of such instruments. Many methods draw upon the somatic symptoms of psychiatric illnesses to identify the diagnosis and quantify severity. A good example is the weight loss commonly associated with depression. These somatic symptoms are frequently manifestations of the physical disorders associated with cancer, particularly when it is advanced. The value of many psychometric questionnaires is therefore limited in cancer patients so those like the Hospital Anxiety and Depression Scale,[17] which seek to avoid the use of somatic symptoms, are especially valuable.

Despite these difficulties, a substantial body of information exists about the psychological disabilities and psychiatric disorders of cancer patients, and the application of measurement methods has been successful in general terms. The availability of useful questionnaires which are relatively independent of somatic symptoms, and have been validated in the context of cancer patients by comparison to more extensive questionnaires, provides the researcher and the cancer physician with valuable tools.

Social problems The social problems for cancer patients are particular and severe compared to the other major life-threatening illnesses. Cancer is our major medical metaphor for evil.[18] It inherited this mantle from infectious diseases such as tuberculosis in the early part of this century and holds its position without challenge. This is most clear in two areas: first, the illness is used as a metaphor for much that is evil within our society. A certain political system may be described as being 'a cancer within our country', and the 'cancerous' role of individual military dictators within their countries has often been quoted; secondly, discussions of cancer often make use of metaphors drawn from the battlefield. There are charities described as 'War on Cancer', patients 'do battle' with their illness, we are all members of 'campaigns', cancers are 'invasive'—and so on. The social implications of being afflicted by a metaphor for evil are inadequately explored, but some manifestations are clear. Cancer patients can become socially isolated at home and in the workplace, with fear of infection used as an excuse for this isolation. Jobs have been lost and families broken by this process which is entirely without substance in any clinical or biological form. Susan Sontag has examined cancer as a metaphor in some detail.[18] A falling incidence of common cancers, which is predicted by epidemiological observations, may not reverse the process of metaphor. Only a reduction in case fatalities can do this, as with tuberculosis, but there is no immediate prospect for a major reduction in case fatalities for common cancers in this century.

Financial disability generated by illness is easy to ignore in the context of busy clinical practice. The cancer patient is not unusual or special in this respect, but his or her well-being may be considerably impaired by frequent hospital visits and loss of career prospects, even if the disease is effectively controlled.

Difficulties related to the treatment

The treatment of most cancers is highly unsatisfactory. Areas of success include complete surgical resection of primary cancer, which is still the main curative treatment modality (eg there is a 30% cure rate in lower gastrointestinal cancers), curative radical radiotherapy for cancer of the cervix or cancers of the head and neck, and curative combination chemotherapy for a small number of relatively uncommon cancers. Apart from its general inadequacy, the hallmark of cancer treatment is its association with deleterious effects upon the patient. In many cases, these are not qualitatively different from those experienced by other patients undergoing, for instance, major surgical procedures. However, in some cases it is possible to characterise the deleterious effects of cancer therapy, and their impact is more severe than that experienced by patients with other life-threatening disorders.

Surgery The degree of damage associated with cancer surgery can vary from straightforward laparotomy with full bowel reconstruction through to major excisions like fore- or hind-quarter amputations. Few other diseases are associated with the more severe range of permanent resection sometimes unavoidable for the cancer patient. In general, there have been striking improvements in the aftermath of surgical procedures for cancer in the last 10 years. Notably, the move from radical to conservative surgery for breast cancer, the availability of reconstructive techniques in the head and neck, microvascular techniques for rebuilding soft tissues in all parts of the body, and the use of prosthetic techniques to replace resected bone, have all greatly reduced the mutilation suffered by patients undergoing cancer operations. However, amputations, mastectomy, laryngeal and pharyngeal resections are still sometimes unavoidable.

Radiotherapy The morbidity caused by radiotherapy may be either acute, in association with inflamed epithelial surfaces, generalised malaise or nausea and vomiting, or chronic, when fibrosis or even malignant change can occur. The most severe of these reactions can usually be avoided by carefully delivered therapy, although a fine balance between toxicity and efficacy is usual.

Chemotherapy Toxicity associated with chemotherapy is well described. Common toxicities include alopecia, nausea and vomiting, and marrow suppression, while less frequent toxicities include cardiac, renal and neurological damage. Patients place nausea and vomiting at the top of their list of acutely identified toxicities. They also give a high priority to hospitalisation and financial burdens associated with recurrent treatments of the kinds commonly employed.

As noted above, discussions about treatment in cancer medicine and surgery are complicated balancing acts between efficacy and toxicity

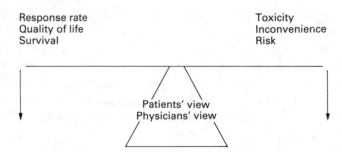

Fig. 1. *The balance between toxicity and efficacy in cancer treatment.*

(Fig. 1). When the treatment is potentially curative in a high proportion of cases, a high level of toxicity may be acceptable, but palliative treatment should not be given unless there is a net improvement in the patients' well-being such that the benefits outweigh the toxicity. In deciding the level of acceptable toxicity for any given probability of remission, both the patients' and the physicians' views should be influential. In good practice, the decision is reached by a process of discussion. Not all patients will manage to resolve a choice about treatment options. Many will ultimately turn to their physician for guidance, at which time it is necessary for the latter to offer clear advice.

Research into the balance of risks and benefits has generally indicated that there are differences between the views of cancer patients, cancer doctors and the general population. In a study by Slevin and colleagues, the level of efficacy perceived to be sufficient to justify a given level of toxicity was evaluated in patients, in the general population and members of the medical and allied professions.[19] Broadly speaking, for patients, moderate toxicity was acceptable in one study for only 1% chance of improvement of their disease, even if that improvement was not curative. The general population were prepared to undergo moderately toxic treatment for quite a small probability of achieving a remission of disease. Doctors (including professional oncologists) were in general less prepared to undergo toxic treatment unless the probability of improvement of their tumour was higher than that expected by both the general population and cancer patients. The interpretation of these observations is complex. It may not be a simple indication that toxic treatment should be given even if there is only a tiny chance of effect, but probably indicates that the decision-taking process must be explored carefully with the patient who should be warned against the dangers of 'grasping at straws'.

In oncology, the issues of 'balance' between toxicity and efficacy are particularly striking. The effect of the illness can be severe in terms both of symptoms and of reduction of life expectancy. The toxicities employed may also be moderate or severe and there may be a risk of treatment-related deaths. In medical specialities, the balance between toxicity and efficacy must be sought, but the immediacy of threat to the patient and the degree of toxicity contemplated may be less than for cancer patients. Measurement of quality of life should be an aid in decision taking in this area, particularly if it is possible to develop instruments which measure quality of life with reasonable reliability and validity and which take on board the complexity of the treatment and disease-related damage that cancer patients may experience.

Possible approaches to measurement

Multiple generic questionnaires

There are now a substantial number of questionnaires capable of either assessing general aspects of dysfunction or behavioural changes in relation to disease (eg the SIP[12] or the Nottingham Health Profile[20]) or more detailed questionnaires which quantify psychiatric morbidity (eg the Present State Examination).[21] These can, and should, be used in cancer patients in detailed studies of disability, distress and emotional disorder, but can have no place in the routine performance of cancer medicine or large-scale cancer clinical trials because of their length and complexity.

Cancer-specific questionnaires

The MRC Cancer Therapy Committee Working Party considered a range of cancer-specific questionnaires and concluded that the Rotterdam Symptom Checklist was probably the present 'best buy'.[15] Since then, further work has been completed, and in some cases reported, on the validation both of the EORTC questionnaire, which has the advantage of offering a range of options related to the specific cancer site, and also of the new analogue scale systems, which are valuable in a research setting when the particular focus of research is quality of life measurement. However, although they are perceived as being quite brief by workers in the quality of life field, they are perceived as lengthy and onerous by many cancer physicians, surgeons and cancer patients. Compliance is often poor, and there is an unwillingness on the part of busy cancer doctors to incorporate them routinely into clinical practice. This is a substantial restriction, and it may be appropriate to consider a trade off between the carefully evaluated questionnaires developed by the research groups and even briefer approaches which can be used in routine practice.

Reductionism and pragmatism

I believe that the measurement of quality of life in cancer patients can be integrated into routine practice in clinical research and clinical service only if the evaluation of quality of life is performed with a very small number of individual questions, perhaps between two and ten. This number of questions might be integrated into the evaluation of the cancer patient in all situations. The junior doctor in outpatients or when 'clerking' a patient into the ward, or the nurse on the ward, could reasonably be expected, or even required, to accumulate information about a small number of facets of a patient's life that might be reasonably uniform and valuable as end-points in clinical trials or in the evaluation of the quality of a service. The ultimate exercise in reductionism would be to a single question about quality of life. However, this would be inadequate because it could not satisfactorily encompass or describe the two major factors identified as independent by the factor analysis reported above: that is, activities of everyday living and emotional well-being. It is not yet clear what might be the gains or losses of a reduced and pragmatic approach to evaluating quality of life. Obvious gains, in terms of brevity, patient and health care worker compliance, and ease of data handling are apparent. How much information is lost when only a small number of questions are used?

This question has been addressed in a study in which quality of life was assessed by using linear analogue scales to ask questions about each of the factors derived from the Toronto quality of life study described above (Fig. 2). In addition, patients completed an overall score for quality of life (Fig. 3). As a further part of this study, they completed the whole questionnaire with 28 items. Multiple regression analysis has been used to assess the relationship between the five individual items and the overall quality of life score in the Uniscale (a full report of this study is to be published[22]). This is clearly a highly stylised system which can allow questions to be asked about the contribution to quality of life scores from each of the five main factors in cancer patient populations. These analyses rely on a number of assumptions, both clinical and statistical. The reliability and validity of the scores have previously been assessed in detail, but the assumptions underlying the construction of the model are of course substantial. Multiple regression methods using the SPSS-X computer programme were used to assess the relationship between the five individual items on the questionnaire and the Uniscale, each of the five items being considered as possible predictors of variation in the Uniscale scores. In the first instance, an analysis was performed using data for all patients.

Please score how *you feel* each of these aspects of your life was affected by *the state of your health*, during *today* (24 hours)

1. To what extent have you been able to carry out your usual daily activities during the last 24 hrs?

Completely .... Normal
unable to   activities
carry out any
activities

2. Symptoms are the unpleasant sensations which an illness produces such as pain, cough, shortness of breath and many others.
   How severe are your symptoms?

Extremely .... No
severe   symptoms

3. To what extent have you felt emotionally distressed or upset (low-spirited, anxious, angry, for instance) as a result of your illness?

Extremely
severely .... Not at all
distressed

4. To what extent have you experienced nausea or vomiting or both during the past 24 hours?

Extremely
severe .... No nausea or
nausea/vomiting   vomiting
or both

5. How far do you feel that your appearance/attractiveness has been altered by your present illness or its treatment?

Extremely
severe .... No alteration
alteration   at all

Fig. 2. *Questionnaire to assess the effect of state of health on various aspects of quality of life in the previous 24 hours.*[22]

Please score how you feel your life has been affected by *the state of your health* (any disease or treatment) during today (24 hours)

My life is .... My life is
extremely   normal
unpleasant   for me with
because of   no changes
the state of   in the state of
my health   my health

Fig. 3. *Questionnaire to assess the effect of state of health on overall quality of life in the previous 24 hours.*[22]

The final model selected had an adjusted coefficient of regression of 0.074—that is, it apparently explained 70.4% of the variation in the Uniscale measurements. (Details of the model are shown in Table 3.) In a range of alternative analyses and models the questions based on the five factors are capable of explaining 58–70% of the variation in the overall quality of life score.[22]

Table 3. Five-item questionnaire—results of regression analysis.

	Individual T-statistic	Individual p-value
Variable selected		
Emotional well-being	9.48	< 0.00005
Activities of everyday living	8.03	< 0.00005
Appearance and attractiveness	4.15	< 0.00005
Symptoms	3.99	0.0001
Variable not selected		
Nausea and vomiting	1.56	0.121

The importance of activities of everyday living and emotional well-being are clearly demonstrated, and would be expected. The relatively small effect of nausea and vomiting upon overall quality of life is surprising, but is consistent throughout the analyses. It may be a real reflection of the importance of nausea and vomiting in our general patient population, but not of their importance in the acute phase after chemotherapy. The questionnaire specifically asked about the previous 24-hour period, and this example enhances the importance which needs to be given to the timing and content of quality of life measurements once the end-points of the study have been identified.

These studies in this very stylised experimental system suggest that a small number of questions carefully directed at the factors which determine quality of life in cancer patients can explain between 50 and 70% of the variation in quality of life. This percentage was not greatly improved when multiple regression was carried out using the 28 items in the original questionnaire. Perhaps this suggests that a small number of questions can explain a great deal of the variance in quality of life, and that asking more questions, although perhaps important in a descriptive way, does not contribute much more information. A proportion of the variation in the quality of people's lives will never be tapped by questionnaires of this kind because it will relate closely to patients' individual interests and priorities.

We would propose that single questions tapping the major factors that determine quality of life in cancer patients are sufficient for most purposes. These appear to be the activities of everyday living, emotional well-being and perhaps appearance/attractiveness. In individual studies or clinical practice it may be important to add items that describe individual areas of great importance. For instance, in an assessment of oesophageal cancer it is appropriate to ask a question about difficulty in swallowing, regardless of what other information may be collected. For most practical purposes, if appropriate descriptive items are included, and questions asked about emotional wellbeing and activities of everyday living, and the answers recorded in a simple quantitative way, no other effort to measure quality of life may be required.

Conclusion

It must be emphasised that this is a preliminary and personal view of the subject. After 10 years of research in this area, the measurement of quality of life in cancer patients has perhaps been explored thoroughly and defined with sufficient precision to allow the sort of information that must be collected in the management of the cancer patient to be chosen carefully and pragmatically. If this is kept to a minimum, it may be possible to integrate it into clinical practice and clinical trials routinely, even if a small amount of information is lost.

References

1. Maguire P, Selby PJ. Assessing quality of life in cancer patients. *British Journal of Cancer* 1989; **60**: 437–40
2. Clark A, Fallowfield LJ. Quality of life measurements in patients with malignant disease: a review. *Journal of the Royal Society of Medicine* 1986; **79**: 165–9
3. De Haes JCJM, van Knippenberg FCE. The quality of life of cancer patients: a review of the literature. *Social Science and Medicine* 1985; **20**: 809–17
4. Fayers PM, Jones DR. Measuring and analysing quality of life in cancer clinical trials. *Statistics in Medicine* 1983; **2**: 429–46
5. Holland JCB, ed. Proceedings of a conference on research methodology in psychological oncology. *Cancer* (suppl) 1984; **53**: 2217
6. McDowell I, Newell C. *Measure health. A guide to rating scales and questionnaires*. Oxford: Oxford University Press, 1987
7. Selby PJ, Robertson B. Measurement of quality of life in patients with cancer. *Cancer Surveys* 1987; **6**: 521–43
8. Ventafridda V, van Dam FSAM, Yancik R, Tamburini M, eds. *Assessment of quality of life and cancer treatment*. Amsterdam: Elsevier, 1986
9. Walker SR, Rosser RM, eds. *Quality of life: assessment and application*. Lancaster: MTP Press, 1988.
10. Tchekmedyian NS, Cella DF. Quality of life in current oncology: practice and research. *Oncology* 1990; **4**: 21–147
11. Selby PJ, Chapman JAW, Etazadi-Amoli J, Dalley D, Boyd NF. The development of a method for assessing the quality of life of cancer patients. *British Journal of Cancer* 1984; **50**: 13–22
12. Bergner M, Bobbit RA, Carter WB, Pollard W, Martin D, Gilson B. The sickness impact profile: development and final reversion of a health status measure. *Medical Care* 1981; **19**: 787–805

13. Gorsuch RL. *Factor analysis*. Philadelphia: Saunders, 1974
14. Bliss JM, Selby PJ, Robertson B, Powles TJ. A method for assessing the quality of life of cancer patients: replication of the factor structure. *British Journal of Cancer* 1992; **65**: 961–6
15. De Haes JCJM, van Knippenberg FCE, Neijt JP. Measuring psychological and physical distress in cancer patients: structure and application of the Rotterdam Symptom Checklist. *British Journal of Cancer* 1990; **62**: 1034–8
16. Schipper H, Clinch J, McMurray A, Levitt M. Measurement of the quality of life of cancer patients: the functional living index — cancer: development and validation. *Journal of Clinical Oncology* 1984; **2**: 472–83
17. Zigmond AS, Snaith RP. The hospital anxiety and depression scale. *Acta Psychiatrica Scandinavica* 1983; **67**: 361–70
18. Sontag S. *Illness as metaphor*. London: Penguin Books, 1983
19. Slevin M, Stubbs L, Plant HJ *et al*. Attitudes to chemotherapy: comparing views of patients with cancer with those of doctors, nurses and the general public. *British Medical Journal* 1990; **300**: 1458–61
20. Hunt S, McEwen J, McKenna S. *Measuring health status*. London: Croom Helm, 1986
21. Wing JK, Nixon J, Mann A, Leff JP. Reliability of the PSE used in a population study. *Psychological Medicine* 1977; **7**: 505–16
22. Bliss JM, Robertson B, Selby PJ (in preparation)

DISCUSSION

Lesley Fallowfield: This chapter is of value insofar as it considers more comprehensively the problems of a specific disease state and how to measure what I define as quality of life, whereas all the previous papers have dealt mainly with the implications of quality-adjusted life years (QALYs), which I think is a completely different agenda.

Peter Selby summarises well some of the validation procedures that need to be gone through when an instrument for a specific disease state is being developed. Trying to hone down such an instrument to a few short questions for routine use by clinicians is a pragmatic solution to an apparent dichotomy currently within medical practice: that quality of life issues are either completely ignored, or patients, researchers and everybody else are over-burdened with lengthy questionnaires that no one has the time, or often the expertise or inclination, to process properly. I agree that a reduced scale may have some value, but only if it were used as a screening tool. There is an analogy here with other aspects of medical practice. If a patient's pulse is thready, weak and irregular, it would suggest to the doctor that perhaps that patient's blood pressure should be measured and an ECG and chest X-ray performed. A first observation leads on to more specific measures. I can accept the use of quality of life type questions in their general sense only if clinicians then go on to use more comprehensive tests for specific areas.

Peter Selby mentioned that the answer to a question about the quality of someone's life depends upon the sort of measure used. The whole area suffers from the inappropriate use of questionnaires called 'quality of life inventories' which were not designed for that purpose. This includes the work of Rachel Rosser and Paul Kind, which has suffered as a consequence. Many of the demands made upon their early work were unreasonable.

Clinicians and patients may have different views about what constitutes quality of life. A measure which has face validity for the former may be irrelevant for a patient in a disease state.

In looking at quality of life, consideration also has to be given to measures needed to help in resource allocation, and also the measures to use if the primary aim is to determine the best treatment between patients. Different sorts of measures would probably be used in clinical trials from those that I would recommend clinicians to use routinely in practice, for example, if they want to determine some sort of management on the basis of results from an inventory. If one of the more comprehensive tools like the Rotterdam Symptom Checklist is used, the responses to single items will suggest appropriate interventions that will help patients. For example, the Rotterdam Symptom Checklist (see Ref. 15) has an item on sexual response. Many cancer patients have inhibited sexual interest and activity, as a result not only of their functional disabilities, but also of their depression and other feelings. If a response to this item reveals problems in this area, a clinician can offer possible interventions, such as counselling, consultation with a liaison psychiatrist and so on.

This is why I prefer a more global approach to measuring quality of life, rather than reducing measures down to simple one-off questions to which there are one-off responses which will not help in terms of available interventions.

We have focused in our discussions very much on the needs of society implied by rationing of resources. The clinician's essential problem, the individual patient under care, has been somewhat forgotten.

Anthony Hopkins: Lesley Fallowfield has pointed out clearly that two different agendas are represented here. Some people are concerned with measures of quality of life which may help in clinical trials for specific diseases, or indeed in individual patient care, by pointing up areas of concern to the patient to which clinicians had not previously been alerted. Using measures of quality of life in this way, however, does not help decisions about allocation of resources to groups of patients with different diseases.

Sonja Hunt: Certain components of existence are intuitively thought of as related to something called 'quality of life', but we are still not sure about their validity. Not enough work has been done. If there was a sounder theoretical and conceptual basis for the work, some agreement might be possible. Perhaps measurements could then be made in different ways, but at least we would know what was being measured. A distinction must be made between what patients and professional people think about the quality of a patient's life.

Peter Selby: Most of the questions in the sorts of questionnaires discussed by Lesley Fallowfield and myself are derived from patients, not doctors. The building bricks that construct the concept of 'quality of life' with which we work come from patients, not health care professionals.

Roy Carr-Hill: Health does not affect quality of life; health *state* affects *health-related* quality of life. We have to be clear about this distinction. There is quality of life, which is everything in the world; there is health-related quality of life, which is how an individual views his own and other people's health; and there is health state which may affect overall quality of life, and perhaps might also affect the individual's view of quality of life elsewhere—all these are different concepts.

Peter Selby: There is no agreed, ideal definition of some global concept of quality of life, and certainly no cross-cultural approach to a definition. It is difficult enough to define health-related quality of life, and we can perhaps define only a small number of minimum dimensions to include within that domain. The current state of research in this field is such that everyone needs to define what he or she is dealing with and what he or she is seeking to measure. It would be splendid if a group of people were to work on the semantic issues of the definition of quality of life.

9 | Quality of life assessments and elderly people

John Grimley Evans

Professor of Geriatric Medicine, Nuffield Department of Geriatric Medicine, Radcliffe Infirmary, Oxford

Introduction

The pursuit of happiness is widely recognised as the main aim of human life. Health is valuable only insofar as it fosters happiness, and longevity only insofar as it offers further opportunities for happiness. The concept of quality of life as a health service outcome measure therefore sounds close to what ought to be the central business of health services. It has been claimed to be particularly suitable as an outcome measure for older people on the assumption that they will be more interested in quality than in length of survival from health interventions. This assumption may be partly an inappropriate projection of younger people's ideas about being old.

Conceptual ambiguities in quality of life assessment

Quality of life has the disadvantage of being a fashionable concept to which everyone feels obliged to pay lip-service. In doing so, they project onto it different aspects of meaning, the accretion of which may lead to its being all things to all men and therefore nothing useful to anybody. Three main lines of investigation have contributed to its parentage.

Psychometric approach

The first is the psychometric approach to the assessment and comparison of states of mind and subjective experience. What is being measured is defined as subjective, so it may be too readily assumed that the methods of measurement and data they produce are non-objective and 'soft'. The hardness of methods lies in such measures as their reliability, validity and sensitivity. Psychometric methods may stand up to investigation of these properties better than many other assessments that provide the basis for important clinical decisions.

Behavioural techniques

The second tradition that has made a major contribution to the development of the concept of quality of life is that of behavioural techniques, notably utility measurement and decision analysis.

It is important to recognise that the psychometric and these other methods are not necessarily measuring the same thing. Indeed, in the few instances in the literature where both methods have been applied to the same situations their correlation is so low as to suggest that they are in fact measuring different things—although more systematic examination of this issue is expected.[1] Perhaps the discrepancies are not surprising. Essentially one approach measures a state of mind, and the other also measures some aspect of value put on that state of mind. Many people feel their quality of life has improved considerably following the imbibition of a couple of dry martinis. It does not follow, however, that they would want to spend all their time in such a state or devote a large proportion of their disposable income to the purchase of the necessary ingredients.

It must also be recognised that utility and decision analysis techniques based on presentation of hypothetical situations have not been formally validated as accurate predictors of the way people make decisions in real-life situations. Validity cannot be assumed from reliability.

Functional variables

The third theme in the parentage of assessment of quality of life has been the measurement of functional variables such as mental function, social status, physical abilities and independence. Various forms of systematic symptom check are also now being included as assessments of quality of life. There are valid reasons for measuring all these, but equating them with quality of life is to give that concept a very different meaning from that reflected in psychometric concepts such as autonomy, morale, self-esteem and life satisfaction. The functional status of a patient is more easily measured or perceived by outside observers, especially professional carers, than is his or her subjective state.

Clinical descriptions illustrate the profound differences in the way older people may rate their quality of life compared with what professional carers would expect.[2] The disjunction between quality of life assessed by these two means presumably underlies the observation that doctors' opinions about a patient's desire for cardiopulmonary resuscitation correlate with 'quality of life' as perceived by the doctor, but the patients' wishes do not.[3] The potential tragedy here is that patients assume that their doctors would be able to give an appropriate proxy decision for them, and a sizeable proportion of older people entering American nursing homes wish this to be done. Even relatives seem ill-equipped to make proxy decisions that would accurately reflect old people's wishes,[4] and again this is most probably because of inadequate perception of subjective quality of life. Significantly, both doctors and patients underestimate old people's wishes for life prolongation. This observation is in keeping with other studies which have shown that older people put generally higher values than expected by younger investigators on life even in states of ill-health.

Hornquist has attempted to synthesise these various accreted aspects of quality of life into an extended concept having six domains each with up to five levels.[5] His approach is intellectually coherent, and a valuable warning of the ambiguities in single-dimension measures of quality of life, but he takes the idea into the realm of research and out of the immediately applicable. Given that the different implications of quality of life measured in its three main traditions are recognised, are there any ways of choosing the most appropriate for various situations involving elderly patients? This issue can be addressed only in the knowledge of the characteristics of later life.

Some relevant characteristics of later life

Embodying even simple measures of quality of life in a useful and rigorous way in outcome assessment presents problems for any age group, but some characteristics of later life render old people particularly susceptible to hazards of the uncritical use of measures of quality of life. These characteristics include:

1. The loss of biological adaptability associated with ageing; older people will be more disturbed, both physiologically and psychologically, by inappropriate management than will young people.
2. The reduction in social adaptability occasioned by loss of wealth (and therefore choice and the power it confers) and by social isolation due to loss of family and friends (with the personalised advocacy these can provide).
3. The cultural gap in changing societies such as our own, so that judgements made by younger people may reflect values alien to the generation in which older people grew up. Older people may also be unfamiliar with concepts and situations that the young regard as presenting no difficulty.

4. A number of ageist prejudices embodied in western societies, lead-
   ing to the assumptions that:
   — the values of older people are necessarily out of date and are
     therefore inferior;
   — older people are necessarily less fit than younger people to make
     judgements;
   — older people are less valuable than younger ones and therefore
     less deserving of attention;
   — the capacity to enjoy the pleasures of life inevitably diminishes as
     individuals grow older.
5. Older people have themselves been imbued with some of these
   ageist prejudices and may be too ready to undervalue themselves or
   to fall in with what they believe to be expected of them. Acquies-
   cence of older people in their lowly social status can also be seen as a
   means of reducing cognitive dissonance.
6. For this reason, and because of reduced adaptability, they will be
   more susceptible to immediate environmental influences. This may
   be reflected in evidence of an age-associated increase in field dependence in cognitive control.
7. Because both intrinsic and extrinsic ageing vary between individuals, the heterogeneity of older people is greater than that among
   younger. This important fact may be obscured in the frequent desig-
   nation of older people as the (presumably homogeneous) 'elderly'.
   There will be greater injustices and inappropriate management if
   the choice of care is based on age-specific averages among older
   people than among younger.

Problems arising from special characteristics of the elderly

Some of the difficulties raised by the factors described above are
technical. It may be suspected that older people will have even more
difficulty with concepts of probability in making decisions than the
young. It is widely thought that older people are more risk-averse than
younger adults, but it is not clear whether this is an ageing or a cohort
effect. Questionnaires and interviews may also have their problems. It
would be predicted, for example, that older people would be more
susceptible than younger people to framing and other field effects in
questionnaires and interviews.[6] Ceiling and floor effects are well
recognised in scales validated in younger people and then used on older
people. Measures that may have been validated in prevalence studies
may prove unexpectedly insensitive in some intervention studies
among older people where only marginal changes can be expected.
This has been noted with two functional scales, the Crichton Royal

Behavioural Rating Scale used in a study of long-term care,[7] and the Barthel Scale in a study of geriatric day hospital care.[8]

More fundamental difficulties with measures of quality of life are conceptual, philosophical and ethical. I have complained elsewhere against those ethicists who present their systems without declaring the ideological assumptions on which they are based.[9] Such people act as societal retroviruses: they hope that what they present authoritatively as the RNA of their ethics will lead to the reproduction in society of the DNA of their underlying ideology. We have long suffered from the endemic diseases of crypto-popery and crypto-marxism. We now face an epidemic of crypto-grocery in a world view as a pervasive market in which the criterion of moral evaluation is the profit of the purveyor rather than the satisfaction of the customer.

It seems only fair to review some general issues about assessment of quality of life affecting elderly people in a way that will declare personal bias and assumptions.

First, specifically in the context of the assessment of well-being, one of the essential properties of the scientific method lies in comparison. The way quality of life is rated will depend on what is seen as the frame of reasonable or attainable alternatives. This reference range will inevitably differ between the old and the young. Older people's tendency to give optimistic estimates of their state of health and well-being perhaps reflects Maurice Chevalier's well-known pronouncement that growing old really is not too bad when you consider the alternative. There are problems here, however. Should old people be allowed to rest in a state with which they report satisfaction but which we know could be improved? If they are content with a lower functional status and are more dependent on others than they need be, do they have a duty to co-operate in improvement? Are we moving towards some concept of a British Standard Aged Person, or more probably, a British Standard Expenditure per Aged Person?

Secondly, much of physical science is concerned with comparisons of different intensities of what is apparently or demonstrably a single dimension, for example, temperature. In biological science, however, the situation is often more complicated. Experimental situations have too many uncontrolled variables, and the functionally infinite replication that would permit the statistical subtraction of the noise they produce is rarely feasible.

In medical science a third level of complexity is added in that our concern may not be with the accurate identification of effects of manipulating a single variable under the conditions of the traditional experimental paradigm of all other things remaining constant, but rather in what happens in real life. This reflection has led, for example, to the distinction between heuristic and pragmatic designs in clinical trials.[10]

A fourth level of difficulty is that the final outcome of our desires may not be a statement issuing from a pragmatic clinical trial of what happens on average, in general, or in the majority of instances, but a prediction of what will most probably happen to a particular patient under particular conditions and at a particular time. This is certainly what patients want from the health service. The paradigm of the single-patient randomised controlled trial is perhaps the *summum bonum* of those who pursue this idea. As a technique, it is of unfortunately limited applicability. Different hypnotics or analgesics may be comparable in such a study, but chemotherapy cannot be compared with placebo or radical mastectomy with tamoxifen.

A fifth difficulty is raised by the spectre of incommensurability, in the sense that we may be betrayed into attempting to measure on the same scale things which cannot validly be brought to a single common scale. This may be a philosophical issue more than a scientific one, in that it depends upon the prior assumptions and definitions. My view is that in approaching decisions that have practical implications for the delivery of health care to British citizens, a duty is imposed upon us by our common citizenship to ensure that our philosophy is congruent with that of British society, and that the professional values we apply are those that British people will expect to be the values of their health services.

In Britain there is no constitution from which to argue the case, but history and the common ground of political argument embody a potentially definable concept of the uniqueness and sanctity of the individual citizen. This is the view that all citizens should have equal status before the law and an equal minimal and sufficient claim on the collective means of life. If such implicit values of traditional English society are accepted, the value of different lives and the states of well-being of different people are necessarily incommensurable. Human life in the English system is primarily and essentially a subjective experience, not just a congeries of objective manifestations. There is therefore no way in which x years of life for Miss A can ethically be brought to a common scale with y years of life for Mr B. If there is an attempt to do this, it is in fact presenting Dr C's view of the life of Miss A and Mr B—which is the assumption that a year of the one is indistinguishable from a year of the other. This is clearly not true, since Miss A or Mr B, not to mention their friends and families, could easily tell the difference.

If this argument smacks of casuistry, some people might prefer the psychometric approach. If life is validly regarded as essentially a subjective experience, Miss A's life can no more be compared with Mr B's than it can be determined whether what Miss A experiences as what she calls 'green' is what Mr B experiences as what he calls 'green'.

The deduction from these arguments is that the ethical basis for the distribution of health resources should be primarily to do good to the greatest number. It may or may not be possible to afford to offer the greatest good, but we should strive to do the most we can. This second constraint may raise issues of timeliness (a patient may be able to wait for a hernia repair but not for cardiac resuscitation), and thus of queueing. As an instrument of social equity, the well-ordered queue has a hallowed place in the British way of life and is not without its ethical virtues.

Assessments of quality of life enable us to offer and to choose between effective treatments for individuals but they should not be used to decide which individuals are treated. Moreover, since individual lives are incommensurable, it follows that their value is non-finite. It is therefore intrinsically improper to treat them as if they were finite, and multiply each by factors such as quality of life or life expectancy. The potential virtues of quality-adjusted life years (QALYs) for helping particular patients to choose between different treatments are enormous. The ethical, technical and philosophical objections to using QALYs to decide which patients are offered treatment are so gross that it is astonishing they have gained such credibility. As several commentators have recognised, it is because QALYs can be used by managers and politicians as an alternative to thought and as a means of denying accountability. It would surely be more healthy socially that resources should be allocated by lottery, as John Harris has suggested,[11] than by confidence trick.

A sixth difficulty could be regarded as a special case of the preceding but raises such particular horrors that it merits specific mention. It is easy to include in our measurement range states evaluated by people with no experience of that state. It has been repeatedly demonstrated that people with particular diseases or undergoing treatments assess their quality of life differently from healthy people asked to guess what it would be like to be in such a situation. The same is seen in the appraisal of old age.

Perhaps the grossest example of unwarrantable measurement is the facile way in which some people, notably health professionals rather than patients (who may feel closer to the implications of the issue), seem ready to categorise some states of health as being worse than death (see the data reported by Williams[12]). It is no business of someone who claims to be an empirical scientist to pretend that he or she knows what being dead feels like. Of course we all know what it *looks* like, and that it has some attractions as an option for some (other) people. After all, economics leaves us in no doubt that dead people are considerably cheaper to support than living ones — a consideration that can easily bias the thinking of managers and clinicians in under-resourced and overstressed health services. Many of us hold beliefs, worship ideals and reach for goals that give logical coherence to comparative valuations of different states of personal well-being for ourselves. In the context of the alleged values of traditional English society, we have no right to make such judgements if they may affect the lives of others, yet how easily we can be manipulated into doing so. It is worrying that there are people who seriously propose that decisions affecting health services should be made on such a basis.

Some practical issues

Measures of quality of life are offered for use in a number of different contexts, some more legitimate than others. My objection to the use of assessments of quality of life to decide who gets treatment has already been raised. Perhaps their ideal use is the presentation to a patient of information about the probable outcomes on multidimensional scales of assessment of different interventions, so that he or she may choose the one that best fits his or her hopes and values. It is only at a significantly lower level of desirability that such information would be used to decide which single treatment will be provided or funded. This is conventional, but may do violence to the principle which, as already emphasised, is particularly relevant to older people, that individuals differ and not everyone would wish to have, or indeed be right to choose, the treatment that gives the best average effects for their sex and age group.

As a prevalence measure, measures of quality of life are of little value, because normative values have been neither established nor shown to be stable. The virtues of measurement of quality of life lie in direct comparisons, preferably within-individual comparisons. Within-individual changes before and after interventions can be compared as outcomes in randomised controlled clinical trials. Techniques involving conventional questionnaires[13] and visual analogue scales[14] have been shown to be applicable to older people. As implied earlier, there should be much more scepticism about applying the more sophisticated techniques of utility and decision analysis to a random selection of the current generation of elderly British people.

Situations may be complex: for example, quality of life as one outcome measure may not be congruent with others. A recent trial of nursing home care against conventional geriatric care showed better quality of life but faster functional deterioration in the nursing home setting.[15] This finding may have increased rather than diminished the uncertainty of administrators about which form of care is preferable.

Another form of complexity is where the changes in measures of quality of life show different trajectories under two different treatments. Comparisons of surgery with chemotherapy for malignant disease may show initial deterioration in quality of life under chemotherapy although ultimately survival may be prolonged. Gelber *et al.* attempted to overcome this problem by computing integral quality-adjusted time without symptoms or toxicity (Q-TWiST).[16] Even this does not demonstrably and entirely solve the problem for older people because of the issue of discounting. Economic models commonly embody a fixed proportional discounting to benefits or costs arising at times in the future. Younger patients may see the future in uniform terms so that higher Q-TWiST scores are attractive whatever the shape of the curve from which such integral values have been obtained. Will this necessarily be true for older people to whom, as individuals, the early toxicity may seem more certain than the later survival? Does an old person see two years as two years or as a percentage of his or her remaining life expectancy? Although in youth we look to the future for the fulfilment that will produce the overall valuation on our lives (many of us with increasing desperation into middle age) it is wrong to assume that in old age we look only to the past and the present. Disengagement theory offered an excuse to society to detach itself from its older members but it is now recognised as a strategy for preventing or dealing with disappointment, not as a recipe for successful ageing. Whether or not the closing horizon is ignored, most old people retain hope, if not confidence, in the future. I am not convinced that the parameters of that hope have yet been analysed sufficiently to understand how the time integrals of quality of life outcomes from health interventions should be evaluated for older patients.

Conclusion

Much remains to be done before the practical and theoretical basis of assessments of quality of life among elderly people can become routine. The first danger in the present situation is that the idea is so fashionable, and some of the uses to which such measurements can be put so attractive to some vested interests, that its use and even its imposition may antecede the necessary proper evaluation. The second danger is that the inevitable disillusionment with inadequately evaluated measurement instruments will lead to the discrediting of the whole approach.

References

1. Tsevat J, Dawson NV, Matchar DB. Assessing quality of life and preferences in the seriously ill using utility theory. *Journal of Clinical Epidemiology* (suppl) 1990; **43**: S73–7

2. Grimley Evans J. The sanctity of life. In: Elford JR, ed. *Medical ethics and elderly people*. Edinburgh: Churchill Livingstone, 1987: 78–92

3. Uhlmann RF, Pearlman RA. Perceived quality of life and preferences for life-sustaining treatment in older adults. *Archives of Internal Medicine* 1991; **151**: 495–7

4. Seckler AB, Meider DE, Mulvihill M, Paris BEC. Substituted judgement: how accurate are proxy predictions? *Annals of Internal Medicine* 1991; **115**: 92–8

5. Hornquist JO. Quality of life: concept and assessment. *Scandinavian Journal of Social Medicine* 1989; **18**: 69–79

6. O'Connor A. Effects of framing and level of probability on patients' preferences for cancer chemotherapy. *Journal of Clinical Epidemiology* 1989; **42**: 119–26

7. Bond J, Gregson BA, Atkinson A. Measurement of outcomes within a randomised controlled trial in the evaluation of the experimental NHS nursing homes. *Age and Ageing* 1989; **18**: 292–302

8. McWilliam J, Brodhurst S, Grimley Evans J. A regional audit of geriatric day hospitals (in preparation)

9. Grimley Evans J. Age and equality. *Annals of the New York Academy of Sciences* 1988; **530**: 118–24

10. Schwartz D, Lellouch J. Explanatory and pragmatic attitudes in therapeutic trials. *Journal of Chronic Diseases* 1967; **20**: 637–48

11. Harris J. QALYfying the value of life. *Journal of Medical Ethics* 1987; **13**: 117–23

12. Williams A. Applications in management. In: Teeling-Smith G, ed. *Measuring health: a practical approach*. Chichester: John Wiley, 1988: 225–43

13. Fletcher AE, Dickinson EJ, Philp I. Audit measures. Quality of life instruments for everyday use with elderly patients. *Age and Ageing* 1992; **21**: 142–50

14. Ebrahim S, Brittis S, Wu A. The valuation of states of ill-health; the impact of age and disability. *Age and Ageing* 1991; **20**: 37–40

15. Bowling A, Formby J, Grant K, Ebrahim S. A randomised controlled trial of nursing home and long-stay geriatric ward care for elderly people. *Age and Ageing* 1991; **20**: 316–24

16. Gelber RD, Goldhirsch A, Cavalli F. Quality-of-life-adjusted evaluation of adjuvant therapies for operable breast cancer. *Annals of Internal Medicine* 1991; **114**: 621–8

DISCUSSION

Astrid Fletcher: John Grimley Evans highlights certain issues in the measurement of quality of life which I do not think are necessarily unique to the elderly but are of particular relevance. Several issues in his paper relating to the use of utilities as a basis of choosing who should be treated have already been discussed, but one that deserves high-lighting is the principle that all life should be given equal weight, and therefore that an elderly life should be valued as highly as a young one. Lip-service is probably paid to this, but it is not borne out in public health interventions. There is some evidence that society does not consider that an elderly life is valued as highly as a child's: the preventive services for the elderly are virtually non-existent, screening for breast and cervical cancer is not offered to women aged over 65, elderly patients are not consistently advised to stop smoking, and cholesterol-lowering diets are not offered to them, despite the poten-tially large benefits because of the high incidence of disease in the elderly.

This chapter also stresses the potential conflicts in the different measurements of quality of life. On the one hand, subjective assess-ments are obtained from the patients—a sort of experience of their lives—and, on the other, there are measurements of function, mostly made by some other person, usually performance-related, and always judgemental, because a score must be given or a function hierarchically measured.

Both approaches are necessary when considering elderly people, although I accept that considerably more information is needed about the disparities between them. I agree with Sonja Hunt and John Grimley Evans that a conceptual model of quality of life in the elderly needs to be developed which is relevant to British society today, and which incorporates the changing attitudes of different cohorts of people as they age. I do not believe that what has been called 'the rocking-chair approach' in considering the quality of life in the elderly, which looks at how the elderly adapt to being old, is a useful approach to continue to take. More objective and subjective data are needed from elderly people to draw attention to some of their problems and needs. Some of the early studies by Peter Townsend on poverty considered issues of concern to people who provide health care for the elderly. For elderly people, the boundaries are blurred between health, the conse-quences of ageing and the effects of the environment in which they live, so distinctions between health-related and other components of quality of life cannot be clearly made.

Most of the relevant outcome data in the elderly relate closely to their quality of life, not just to ignoring the benefits which might occur in terms of life expectancy. I also think that survival—extension of life—is important for elderly people. We may think of the very large number of procedures or health care interventions that have been tried in the elderly without proper study, with absolutely no evidence or very dubious evidence of benefit, and the enormous costs and consequences for resource allocation that have come out of haphazard decision-making. The most obvious example is the requirement of the National Health Service and Community Care Act (1990) that general practitioners provide annual health checks for those aged over 75—a requirement that has a huge resource implication for family doctors. This decision was based on virtually no data. There are three small randomised controlled trials, one of which has mortality as an outcome measure, but with insufficient numbers for adequate power. None of the three trials considered some measures of quality of life as an outcome measure of the effectiveness of annual health checks.

There are numerous examples in the geriatric medicine literature of assessments and interventions in elderly people being haphazardly implemented and equally haphazardly taken away. Day hospitals were brought into being with great enthusiasm 20 years ago, and are now disappearing at about the same speed as they were implemented. There is only one randomised control trial of which I am aware (not in this country) which even attempted to measure the effects of day hospitals upon quality of life. Instead of spending a lot of time and resources in trying to devise a perfect health index, far more should be spent in assessing some of the important everyday deliveries of health care in the elderly.

Alan Williams: In this discussion we have been asked to develop a philosophically well-grounded conceptual model of quality of life. Philosophers have been struggling with this problem for thousands of years, and it will not be solved in the next 1,000 years. Is it not sufficient to try to work in a particular context with the main characteristics that people value, although everything they value may not be considered? Is this sufficient as a way forward, or do we have to cease work for another 5,000 years until a conceptual basis has been sorted out?

Roy Carr-Hill: Alan Williams is arguing that some kind of measurement is better than none, but the question is *who* should be making the judgements about resource allocations between different types of treatment and health care intervention by health professionals? I argue that this will not be answered by getting a large number of responses to questionnaires, even going through all the statistical hoops with them. This is not the right way to study this problem because there would have been all kinds of 'intervention' in terms of the construction of the questionnaire. Even if it can be accepted that the way in which people react to these questionnaires is understood, this is still not a democratic way to provide data for resource allocation. The task has to be done, not by economists in conjunction with doctors, but by the public, and I do not deny that it will take a long time.

Lesley Fallowfield: When doctors, nurses, patients and their primary carers and supporters all fill in the same questionnaire on functional status, quality of life, emotional well-being and so forth, nearly every study has shown poor correlation between the different respondent groups. It is important to involve other people in constructing the questionnaires. Also, as far as possible, the patient should fill in any questionnaire and not the primary carer who may give prejudicial assessments of a patient's status. A doctor's view of the quality of life of an individual may sometimes be accurate, but often is not.

Nick Ross: In essence, Roy Carr-Hill is stating that Alan Williams' instrument should not be introduced because it does not have a methodological basis on which everyone can agree, it can be seen to be counter-intuitive, and it may not reflect democratic principles. We live in a deeply flawed and imperfect world in which difficult decisions are made about the provision of medical resources. It may well be that QALYs are not yet fully thought through, but at least they are an attempt to introduce some systematic basis into what, at the moment, is utterly unsystematic. I do not agree with the view that until we get a perfect system we should not have it at all. We have a flawed system at present in which decisions are being made. We should begin to introduce into it some systematic process, and try to refine it.

Sonja Hunt: We are still not discussing the issue of whether QALYs are a good basis for making these decisions, which is really the question to address. There may well be better bases.

Roy Carr-Hill: I am saying that there are no technical grounds for supposing that QALYs provide any better basis for resource allocation than arbitrary 'shroud waving'.

10 | Ethical issues arising from measures of the quality of life

Sir Douglas Black
Past President, Royal College of Physicians

Introduction

I am no expert on the different methods of measurement of quality of life, so I will leave techniques to the experts and confine my paper to the *use* of such measurements.

First, I shall sketch an ethical framework which may be considered appropriate to health service problems, and then consider the ethical aspects of using measures of quality of life as part of the assessment of outcome.

An ethical framework

Taking great care at this stage not to define what is 'good' and what is 'evil', let me postulate that the question which lies at the heart of ethical or moral discourse, and without which such discourse would be impossible, is why should we do good rather than evil? The answers which have been suggested to this question are many and varied, but they fall into two main groups: the deontological and the consequentialist.

The deontological position

The *deontological* position, of which Immanuel Kant is the great exponent, postulates a supreme moral law which prescribes for our conduct a number of categorical imperatives, the character of which is such that they would be generally accepted, at least in principle, and which imply that people should always be treated as ends and not as means. A difficulty inherent in the deontological position is the source or justification of the 'supreme moral law' itself. As Raanan Gillon has pointed out, the word deontological stems from the Greek *deon* (duty), not from the Latin *deus* (god).[1] The term thus does not imply a theistic basis for moral conduct, nor of course does it exclude it. 'Sweet are the uses of ambiguity', to misquote the melancholy Jaques. Belief in a moral law, however derived, is pragmatically a stimulus to good conduct, and it provides an acceptable explanation of why many people 'do good'. It is distinctly less powerful, however, as an explanation of why other people, or indeed the same people at other times, 'do evil', and the subjective perception of moral law is not open to objective observation as are the consequences of our behaviour.

The consequentialist position

It may be in part this last consideration, the subjectivity of moral law, which stimulated philosophers such as John Stuart Mill to adopt the utilitarian approach, which grounds good ethical action in a desire for good consequences, among which happiness was stressed by Bentham, and before him by Francis Hutcheson in 1725:

> That action is best which procures the greatest happiness for the greatest numbers.

This *consequentialist* position has the considerable strength that consequences, unlike motives, are accessible to observation and assessment: what happens is visible, what prompts is occult. There are, however, difficulties. For any complex course of action, perception and analysis of consequences are likely to be limited to those clearly linked to it, and which follow soon after it. In its hedonist variant, the question arises of *whose* happiness—A is happy, B is not—a difficulty that is surely compounded should we move from the individual to the group.

Ethical principles

In relation to practical affairs, a purely pragmatic approach would, I believe, lean towards the consequentialist position, probably with no explicit formulation or recognition of the ethical basis of action but with an alert eye to those consequences which can be anticipated. This no doubt suffices in most situations, but is less than adequate when the consequences are uncertain or when there are competing interests. My own belief, sometimes summarised in the phrase 'situation ethics', is that the specific features of the clinical or administrative situation must be the dominant factors in making the decision(s).[2] These can be assisted by having regard to ethical principles, not of such generality as moral law or pure utility, but more derivative in the sense of being closer to reality and application. Examples of such principles are:

— *respect for autonomy*, the modern phrasing of the Kantian principle that individuals must be treated as ends not as means, and it implies, among other things, telling the truth and keeping confidential what should be so kept:

— *beneficence* denotes our duty to 'do good' to people which, in the light of the first principle, should be good as perceived by them;
— *non-maleficence* recognises our duty not to do harm to others, even when we are doing good to a patient or client;
— *justice* is the principle of fairness or even-handedness in the face of conflicting interests, which may even include benefit to one at cost to another, or to society at cost to individuals.

In my view, these are not absolute principles, as may be illustrated in two ways. First, taking the principle of autonomy and, within that, the duty of confidentiality, what may be described as *legitimate exceptions* come to mind—I doubt whether many people would hesitate to divulge such health information as might identify the perpetrator of murder or prevent a terrorist attack in a public place. Also, in spite of current fashion, I have yet to be convinced that the whole and unexceptioned duty of a doctor is to tell the whole truth at all times. I would attempt to justify this sad lapse into paternalism (a term almost as opprobrious as judgmentalism), by an appeal to the principle of beneficence. Were the plea to be accepted, it could be my first example of *conflict between principles*, which is my second reason for not considering such principles as absolute. Other examples are conflict between the autonomy of an infected individual and the need to protect others (non-maleficence), and rationing expensive resources (justice?), thus failing in beneficence.

Quality of life

According to Bill Shankly, football is not a matter of life and death—it is far more important than that. In certain clinical situations, the same might be said of 'quality of life', 'well-being', or 'health'—terms we think we understand until we try to define them. It would be crass to suppose that our medical forebears took no account of that dimension when making decisions, but there are features of present-day medicine which make it more important than ever before to consider quality of life—and other aspects which make that consideration more difficult ethically.

Although there are still all too many situations in which medicine is powerless, there is also an increasing number in which medicine or surgery can be critically effective, with great gain both in survival and in well-being. These gains carry a cost, however, both because survival may be achieved without adequate well-being, and because the potent procedures and medications required in the management of desperate illness can themselves, through their side-effects, impair the quality of life. There are, for example, clear possibilities that patients with, say, advanced tumours may be kept alive in a state which is 'worse than death', and that for others, the cure, even if well designed, may turn out to be worse than the disease. The conclusion must be that consideration of quality of life as well as of survival, always implicit in good clinical practice, is more than ever important, and that serious attention must be given to ways of making it explicit.

Let us therefore try to address two difficult questions, each with an ethical component:

1. Is individual quality of life open to quantitative assessment?
2. Can aggregated indices of quality of individual life be used as a component in deciding health services priorities?

Individual quality of life

Informal assessment of consequent quality of life must always have been a component in clinical decision making and, as indicated above, the changes in medical practice make such an assessment more, not less, important and also more difficult. It is more important because there are greater possibilities of influencing the situation for good or ill, and more difficult because of the complexity of what constitutes quality of life, and also because of the emergence of states, previously unknown, such as prolonged coma or medicated survival in high dependency.

As an exercise in demonstrating the complexity of the problems, but also in clarifying them, I acknowledge my debt to Lesley Fallowfield's book.[3] Quality of life is shown to be multidimensional, and also greatly influenced both by the current clinical state and by the previous make-up and situation of the individual.

The dimensions of quality of life include not only the physical condition of the patient, important though this is, but also how he feels about life and his relation to it, how he relates to the social environment, and his capacity to continue working — not the least determinant of that elusive virtue, contentment. Although these matters are not independent variables, they are all worth taking into account in assessing quality of life. It may be worth giving a view on what is ethically desirable in choosing between them. Three possible criteria may be suggested, giving them here in dogmatic form:

1. Assessments made by sufferers from particular states are to be preferred to vicarious estimates. (In the phrase, *experto crede*, the 'expert' in the subjective context of illness is the patient, not the doctor or even the nurse.)

2. A method which takes account of several variables is preferable to uni- or bi-dimensional methods, even at the expense of numerical complexity.
3. When several variables have been measured, some weighting should be made in favour of those which can be more rather than less objectively measured. Table 1 shows how fitness for work may be used in comparing the efficacy of different treatments for chronic renal failure.[4] Although fitness for work combines the physical and psychological dimensions, as well as previous occupation and social opportunity, it is to be criticised as only a single measure—but one not devoid of practicality.

Table 1. Terminal renal failure: fitness for work after different methods of treatment.[4] The horizontal rows give for each method of treatment the probability (p) of the outcome specified at the top of the corresponding column. The final row gives an estimate of the utility (u) of each of the outcomes.

Method of treatment	Degree of employment				Relative value (Σpu)
	Full-time	Part-time	Unemployed	Unfit	
Dialysis					
Hospital	0.34	0.25	0.21	0.20	0.54
Home	0.64	0.16	0.14	0.06	0.74
Transplant					
Live-donor	0.75	0.10	0.10	0.05	0.77
Cadaver	0.66	0.12	0.13	0.09	0.71
Estimated utility	0.90	0.60	0.30	0.10	

The relative value of each of the methods is the sum of the probability of each outcome, multiplied by the outcome's utility; for example, for hospital dialysis, the relative value is: $(0.34 \times 0.9) + (0.25 \times 0.6) + (0.21 \times 0.3) + (0.20 \times 0.1) = 0.54$. Such calculations of value are sensitive to the assessment of utility.

Validity of aggregated measures of quality of life

It is clear that progress has been, is being, and will continue to be made in improving assessment of quality of life in a particular person in a specified clinical situation. A somewhat different question, also with an ethical dimension, stems from any proposal to aggregate this type of information, whether to assess different modes of treatment or to contribute to decisions on the allocation of resources.

There should, in my view, be no hesitation as to the desirability of making judgements, whether they be between treatments or between health service priorities, on as objective a basis as possible and, wherever possible, based on valid numerical data. Where objection has been taken to this, it has usually been on one of two grounds: the inherent difficulty in aggregating data of this nature, and the possibility of systematic bias against groups disadvantaged from causes not related to specific illness. The first objection would apply both to 'clinical' and to 'managerial' applications of the quality of life approach, and the second mainly, if not entirely, to managerial applications.

Difficulty in aggregation arises from the sheer 'untidiness' of figures derived from patients who resemble each other only in sharing a particular clinical predicament, and who differ in myriad ways, not only in the intensity of their individual episode of illness but often more importantly in their attitude to it, their degree of support, previous life-style and social setting. I do not share this first objection. These are the very difficulties which the methods of statistics applied to biology were specifically designed to solve—and have indeed done so in areas of comparable intrinsic complexity.

I have more of a problem with the second objection. I do not quarrel with the principle that one component of 'fairness' lies in the matching of resources to need, and another in using resources to produce optimum outcomes, in groups as well as in individuals. My concern is more fundamental and is derived from the perception that illnesses and their treatment make up only a small part of our fate, which is much more determined by our heredity, age and sex, upbringing and social environment.

My own bias is to allot top priority to children, both for the present and the future. This does not, however, prevent me realising that the elderly also have their needs and that, through no fault of their own, the outcomes of their illnesses are likely to be less favourable than in the young. Similarly, an outcome-based analysis would favour the rich at the expense of the poor, because the latter have conspicuously worse intrinsic health. I am sure that these are not the intentions of advocates of the quality of outcome approach, but when has there ever been an exact match of intention and result?

References

1. Gillon R. *Philosophical medical ethics*. Chichester: Wiley Medical, 1985
2. Black D. Iconoclastic ethics. *Journal of Medical Ethics* 1984; **10**: 179–82
3. Fallowfield L. *The quality of life: the missing measurement in health care*. London: Souvenir Press, 1990
4. Black D. Paying for health. *Journal of Medical Ethics* 1991; **17**: 117–23

DISCUSSION

Michael Lockwood: I want to comment on the extent to which quality and length of life can be brought together in a meaningful way. Irrespective of the methodological strengths or weaknesses of any particular approach, there ought to be ways of combining these two measures because the right way of looking at a life is as a kind of container of things we value. Rationally life should not be valued for its own sake, but for what we can do with or make of it. We need to live in order to do and experience the things we want. There is thus a sense in which quality of life is all that matters: a longer life of a given positive quality is better insofar as it means the enjoyment of *more* of that quality.

Trading off length of life against quality of life is, in principle, no more problematic than, say, when faced with a choice of holidays, deciding whether to spend one week in Crete or two weeks in Torquay. The individual has to decide in which place he will get more of what he hopes to get out of a holiday. I do not mean to trivialise an obviously deeply serious issue, but I would suggest that the logic is essentially the same.

I have no doubt that the ethical principles cited by Douglas Black, of respect for autonomy, beneficence, non-maleficence and justice are excellent—and I dare say I use them myself—but it is not clear to me how these principles are supposed to help, as he suggests, where the consequences are uncertain or there are competing interests. To the extent that neither the likely consequences of our actions nor how to adjudicate between competing interests are known, we do not know what to do.

These principles will not make that uncertainty go away. The role of the principles is, in the main, to focus attention on the different sorts of consequences and competing interests that may be at stake, and to remind us of their ethical significance. How much do the patient or other affected parties stand to gain from a given treatment (beneficence)? How great are the risks of harm (non-maleficence)? To what extent is the patient's autonomy respected in acting in a particular way and, where there are competing interests, what constitutes a just resolution of the conflict?

These principles serve more to raise certain sorts of question than to provide ready-made answers. It would be odd—an extraordinary gift from God—if there were some set of considerations which, for any situation, would indicate, regardless of the factual uncertainties, the best action to take. Life can never be like that.

I agree with Nick Ross (page 119) in querying how much force criticism of a particular methodology of assessing quality of life and so forth has in circumstances in which it is not clear that there is any better methodology on offer. The challenge facing those who argue strenuously against the quality-adjusted life year (QALY) approach to medical resource allocation is to make out a case that the mixture of hunch, habit, prejudice and *ad hoc* expediency that currently underlies much decision making in this area is better than the approach offered by advocates of QALYs.

Nevertheless, any philosopher who encounters the QALY approach will realise at once that it is vulnerable to many of the objections facing classical utilitarianism. The difficulty with aiming simply at maximising QALYs—assuming for the sake of argument that a satisfactory way of measuring quality of life has been achieved—is that such an approach is largely insensitive to considerations of distributive justice. For example, maximising QALYs in regard to treatment designed to extend life would imply discriminating against patients or groups of patients suffering from other health-related distress or disability, even where that had no bearing on the likely effectiveness of the treatment under consideration, since extra years of life for these people would count for fewer QALYs. It hardly seems fair though that patients who are already suffering in other respects should, *for that very reason*, be denied potentially life-saving treatment.

Douglas Black first raised in discussion the question whether QALYs are inherently unfair to the elderly. First, the QALY arithmetic will give higher priority, as regards life-extending or life-enhancing treatment, to those patients whose post-treatment life expectancy is greater, which will obviously tend to favour the young. Secondly, as regards life-extending treatment, higher priority will be given to those patients whose post-treatment quality of life is higher. Elderly patients are thus again liable to lose out, insofar as they are more likely to be suffering from such conditions as arthritis, and the other forms of disability apt to affect people in later life.

Nevertheless, I think the charge of 'ageism' is ill-founded. Consider a hypothetical example in which there are two rival contenders for dialysis, one of whom is 20 years younger than the other but, for reasons unconnected with his need for dialysis, he has a life expectancy comparable to that of the older patient. Let us assume that the two patients can expect a similar post-treatment quality of life. In these circumstances, the QALY-maximisation approach, or indeed any simple-minded utilitarian approach, will say that it is a matter of indifference which of the two patients gets the treatment. The likely gain, in terms of QALYs, will be the same. However, in terms of justice, I think a strong case can be made for favouring the younger over the older patient. The latter, by definition, has already enjoyed more years of life than the younger patient to whom it is therefore surely more equitable to give life-extending treatment. This line of thought, known as the 'fair innings' argument, suggests that, from the point of view of simple justice, far from being objectionably ageist, the QALY-maximisation approach is less sensitive to considerations of age than it ought to be. To this extent, I agree with Douglas Black that age should be taken into account in the setting of medical priorities.

John Grimley Evans: The fair innings argument has been criticised by John Harries, among others. In terms of equity, my view is that the fairness of an innings depends mainly upon the quality of the bowling! It is a pity that our discussion has focused so much on QALYs. The duration element in QALYs confuses and distracts attention from important issues about quality of life assessment in general.

Alan Williams: If we are to decide what is a fair system of distribution in health care, the best experiment is to imagine that we are looking at our society from the outside, and ask within what sort of rules we would want this society to operate if we had no idea of our own place in it. Having carefully thought through this set of rules, lots can then be drawn—and we will find ourselves somewhere in that society. At the level of thought, this is the most promising way to fight our way through the issue of whether we have the right to make judgements upon the lives of other people. Society has to make such judgements; it is no good pretending that an individual clinician or anyone else can avoid them. For example, once it is decided to commit home help to one elderly person, a decision has also been made not to give it to some other person. Some judgement must have been made that this home help would be more useful to person A than to person B. There is no escape, and therefore we have to think how best to make such decisions.

11 | Are measures of the quality of life likely to be useful instruments of social policy?

Howard Glennerster
Professor of Social Administration, London School of Economics

Introduction

Only a combination of the medical and economics professions would probably have been sufficiently arrogant to claim that they were able to produce a measure of the quality of life that would be sufficiently robust to use to allocate resources in the National Health Service (NHS) or elsewhere. Such arrogance derives, however, not only from the nature of these professions and their training but also from the organisational imperatives that face the NHS and, in differing degrees, all the social services. As a colleague once put it, 'Social policy is deeply and essentially paternalistic'.

Rationing of services

When a society has decided to finance services like health collectively and has abjured both price and the ability to pay as the ultimate rationing devices, administrative means to ration resources have to be invented. *Social administration* may be defined as the study of resource allocation in non-market systems, and *social policy* as the study of the boundaries drawn between collective and private provision, and between formal and informal systems of care.

Thus, rationing is a necessary feature of social policy. It can, however, take many forms:
— allocations of revenue or capital expenditure;
— manpower allocations, like limits on places in medical school or consultant posts; and most obviously,
— the rationing of doctors' and social workers' time, putting priorities on access to these scarce professional people.

It is helpful to think of services being rationed in at least two dimensions: first, there is the locus of the rationing decision, which may lie at the highest or most centralised position. I would define this as a Cabinet decision; for example, to allocate so much to health or education. Subsequent decisions are taken at regional or district level, but some of the most important decisions in all social services are taken at the bottom, in the day-to-day judgements made by clinicians, teachers and social workers.

Secondly, there is the nature of the criteria used to make resource decisions, their explicitness and openness—what I call the explicit/implicit dimension (Fig. 1). Traditionally, much social service rationing has been undertaken at the implicit end of the spectrum. Priorities have been unclear, and judgements reached in private according to professional criteria that were never open to debate. Budgets were rolled forward or back according to past allocations (that is, incremental budgeting).

This is all changing fast now, not only in the health service or as a result of the NHS and Community Care Act but as part of a much longer process. Revenue allocations shifted upwards and to the left-hand quadrant of my rationing map with the coming of the Resource Allocation Working Party (RAWP) and the programme budget system (PBS) in the mid 1970s. Contracting is only the logical extension of this process further down the allocative chain. Exactly the same kind of process is underway in the personal social services. Given resource constraints and the growing awareness of the issues by the wider public, it seems to me that explicit rationing—a move from right to left across the map—is bound to happen at all levels and in all social services.

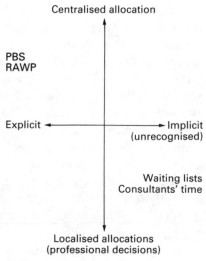

Fig. 1. *A rationing map for the health and social services.*

This process requires open explicit criteria to be available and used in measurement at each stage of the rationing process:

— in the initial resource allocation process to the service unit or professional concerned;
— in the informed decisions made by clinicians and other professionals about their use of those resources;
— in evaluating afterwards the impact of the resources on patient or client outcomes.

It is in this broader context that the use of quality of life measures has to be discussed, whatever the arrogance they seem to display—but also coloured with a large degree of humility. The need for organisations to have some measures at all costs is no justification for presenting them either with bad ones or with measures that cloud the openness and explicitness that I claim to be necessary.

Some general precepts

1. *The more important the quality of life to the final decision the less rationing should be in the hands of the administrator or professional.*

In any area but medical or social care, few people in this country would dream of saying, at least in public, that their chosen way of life is superior to somebody else's—and, what is more, they will force that person to adopt their way of life. When doctors urge us to stop smoking or to drink sensibly they are implicitly saying that a long dull life is better than a short fun-packed drunken one. Fortunately, it is still for us to decide, and clearly the British have different ideas about this from the Americans or people in other countries—and the Scots from the English.

What constitutes a good old people's or children's home? Clearly, if these decisions are to be made collectively, some sensitive measures of quality are needed. Excellent progress is being made, for example, in homes for those with learning difficulties in work by Norma Raynes at Manchester and York. This provides some handle to evaluate the relative quality of care and its relation to costs.

The fundamental question is, however, whether decisions about which residential home is best have to be taken by administrative means. The quality of life in a home, and the aspects of it that are given most importance, are highly person- or family-specific. Might it not be better to give the family a voucher or a cash-limited choice of home or domestic support? Quality of life measures are so often conceived of as purely individualised, whereas in fact the quality of life is a complex mix of factors that includes relationships with other members of the family, partners or residents. These kinds of judgement can be made only by the family or carer and the individual concerned.

There may be many decisions which cannot easily be left to patients or relatives. I am currently carrying out a study of general practice fundholding. One of the objections to this feature of the NHS reforms raised by many district managers is that it prevents them from making consistent judgements about priorities across a district. Fundholders interviewed argued that they are in a much better position than district managers or community physicians to make such decisions because they have much more social and contextual knowledge about individual cases, and can discuss issues with patients. They are essentially arguing, although implicitly, that the combination of preferences that emerge from such an interplay with patients, and their need to keep within the budget constraint, will produce a better guide to priorities than any overall set of priorities derived from a quality-adjusted life year (QALY) table. It is certainly interesting that the kinds of factors that feature in their contracts are somewhat different to those that feature in the contracts of their districts. Patient convenience is higher up their order of priorities, as is speed of treatment compared to distance travelled.

In short, quality of life measures may be necessary to inform some strategic or professional rationing decisions, but the more consumer choice that can be substituted the better.

2. *Different dimensions of the quality and length of life should not be conflated.*

The argument here is similar to that in the wider planning and cost-benefit literature. Is it really meaningful to conflate measures of the cost of road building, environmental damage to Norman churches and lost travel time into one measure — that is, money? The attractiveness of it is that it gives a simple decision criterion, but the problem is that it counts apples and elephants, when apples are traded and elephants are not. How meaningful are the trade offs between length of life and pain, taken by anonymous others in an unreal situation? The issues have been admirably argued by Roy Carr-Hill[1] and at this workshop, and there is no need to elaborate them further.

Many environmental planners concluded from their somewhat similar debate a decade ago that it was better to keep the dimensions separate: to measure the impact both on the environment and on travel time, and ask people to do their own trade offs between time saved for a million passengers and the loss of the church and the cost of an alternative route. The same conclusion applied to the quality of life debate would mean keeping the different aspects of 'quality' and 'quantity' in different columns, as it were.

The impact of different spending choices on functional impairment could be measured separately and decision takers asked to test the possible trade offs. One investment may increase the number of lives lived, but may also increase the number of severely disabled people; another would increase the mobility of so many thousand people. Such a presentation makes life more difficult for those who have to take decisions because they are not faced with one apparently unambiguous choice. It does bring out, however, rather than hide, the value judgements inherent in the choices. The same kind of considerations apply, I believe, to a whole range of efficiency and equity issues in social policy.

3. Multiple indicators should be used, not just health measures.

There is a great danger in confining this discussion to QALYS and individualised measures of health. Clearly, the quality of life is more than this. Do disabled people competing in the Olympics for the disabled derive more or less pleasure from the experience than 'normal' athletes? A glance at television suggests it is more. To many, the companionship derived from shared difficulty has been a life-enhancing experience. It is highly misleading to judge the experience of someone in a home only by the physical surroundings or even by the attitudes of the staff. A person's social network, links with the family and so on may be far more important to that person.

Measuring social health in terms of social interaction, where it is desired, social support, psychological well-being, life satisfaction and morale, are all basic ingredients in any discussion on quality of life. Ann Bowling has reviewed the range of instruments that exist.[2] They should be included in the range of outcomes being weighed.

4. Indicators should be used as a basis for public discussion not private executive action.

The choices inherent in the rationing decisions that have to be made in the health field are political dynamite, and the natural response of both clinicians and managers is to retreat into private session and settle the issues without the distress of public debate. Increasingly, this option will not be open. The distance between the caring professions and the public is narrowing fast. It may still be evident for the medical profession, but not for long, and has already disappeared for the social work profession. Our social workers have to be taught how to cope under the spotlight of public scrutiny, and the medical profession will have to do the same. Thus, openness and consistency will be forced on the professions and on the rationers of resources. This will force some ugly debates into the open, such as what priority should be given to AIDS patients, and will the disabled and the mentally ill gain or lose? What will such open debate do for the pressure to spend more on the NHS?

References

1. Carr-Hill RA. *The QALY industry: can and should we combine morbidity and mortality into a single index?* York: Centre for Health Economics, 1988
2. Bowling A. *Measuring health: a review of quality of life scales.* Milton Keynes: Open University Press, 1991

General discussion

Alan Williams: First, the general criticism of QALYs—which I am sure is true—is that at a technical level we could do much better than we have done so far. The second suggestion is that there are better validated and more reliable instruments for measuring quality of life than those so far used. If there are any such instruments, I would like to hear about them. Thirdly, openness and transparency apply to research as well as to policy. All our data, apart from the Euroqol© data (which will soon be included), have been lodged with the Economic and Social Research Council (ESRC) survey research archive and are available for general use.

Astrid Fletcher: In most of our discussion the view has been taken that there is no alternative to QALYs and that they are the best research tool on offer at the moment. This is not true: it is already known to some extent how to make decisions, for example, in hypertension, about whom to treat, and the best benefits in terms of risk. These kinds of decisions are not made by combining measures of quality of life and life expectancy but by taking overviews of results of trials, looking at the effects of quality of life on treatment, the relative effects of different treatments of hypertension on myocardial infarction and so on. A range of decision-making areas is considered when ordinary physicians decide which hypertensive patients to treat, and what levels of blood pressure to treat and to aim for. There is a danger in the argument that everything has to be simple, that it will be better than what is being done at the moment, which is uninformed.

Jack Dowie: As soon as a researcher develops something simple, people will say that it is too simple, but when research workers add three or four dimensions, people will say that the proposal has 'Ptolemaic complexity' (page 89). It is a no-win situation as soon as we move from the sacred ground that the *status quo* is all right, and that well-meaning, sensible men and women in their private offices are capable of taking all these difficult decisions. QALYs are about taking account of things because this is the only way in which true openness, explicitness and accountability can exist.

I have identified a new disease. The sufferers can be identified as people who are able quite well to diagnose defects in the existing way of doing things, and will even admit to some imperfections in themselves. However, they instantly become unable to see those defects—which in fact disappear completely—as soon as an alternative way of tackling the problems or remedying the defects is suggested. The onset is particularly rapid if the alternative involves numbers or equations— and, of course, instantaneous if it involves any reduction in income or increase in workload.

I want to launch a campaign which I have called CHANCE, or Campaign to Hinder the Advance of Non-comparative Evaluation, because what we have been discussing here is essentially non-comparative evaluation. Nobody is advancing QALYs, or a variety of QALYs, as a perfect solution to anything. They will be hopelessly inadequate as a measure for allocating resources. The only issue is whether a QALY-type method is *better* than some other method of allocating existing resources because the absolute is not attainable.

Martin Buxton: If it is agreed that the ethical basis of allocating resources should be to do good to the greatest number (as proposed by John Grimley Evans in Chapter 9), the QALY framework is no help. Cost per QALY analysis presumes an objective of maximising the 'good' done to society as a whole. This seems to me to be a much more reasonable objective although I, like others, would recognise that this maximisation of total health benefit within a given budget (maximising the number of QALYs achieved) has to be subject to some equity constraint ensuring that all receive an acceptable minimum level of provision, given their particular needs.

Roy Carr-Hill: There are many assumptions in the literature about QALYs and about the aims of the health service, but I believe these aims are unclear. For example, the role of carers has been discussed—an example of issues not really addressed by QALYs.

Clive Smee: I hope that the publication of *The health of the nation* will promote a discussion of the ultimate ends of the health service. The key areas for which targets are set will provide some information.

Peter Selby: I defend the clinical decision-taking process. In the practice of oncology, for example, there are consensus guidelines for most areas of technical day-to-day practice. These are arrived at by open discussion, to which patients, nurses and others contribute. There is also the process of audit, which ensures that the practice of medicine is examined by independent people from other teams and other specialties.

Sally Macintyre: Paul Walker stated (Chapter 5, discussion) that his health authority likes QALYs because they avoid the need to think. It is a serious situation if the use of these measures means that people do not have to think about what they are doing and why.

Participants were asked to indicate to what uses measures of quality of life were being currently put.

Christopher Pollitt: I suspect that none of us knows what use is presently made of QALY data. My hunch is that they are being used in a spasmodic *ad hoc* way by some health authorities where there is somebody with an interest in them, who at least reads some of the literature, and is prepared to take the risk of pushing this kind of data into the flow of decisions. It may be that QALYs are being used to support existing prejudices.

Clive Smee: People from all levels, from district health authorities through regions up to civil servants in this country and in other national governments from Australia to the USA, have been asking for some years now what is known about the cost per QALY of particular treatments. If we, as officials, are asked what is known about the cost-effectiveness of particular interventions, should we say we know nothing, when in fact there is some information? Senior officials and Ministers are well aware of the weaknesses and doubts that surround this whole area.

Paul Walker: My experience is that the factual information that influences a decision at district or regional level is minimal, and what I call 'political content' has been all dominating.

Rachel Rosser: My experience is slightly different. I tend to get called in when people are either considering using the QALY technique or have started to use it and are rather worried about the initial results, often justifiably. I try to explain that we are working towards some quantitative information, as accurate as possible, which would help people to think. There is a limit to the amount of time, mental energy and background reading that any group of people can spend in decision making. The idea is to stimulate these other discussions, particularly ethical discussion. For example, one problem with the present valuations is that the highest number of QALYs is obtained by giving most treatment to the least ill people. What happens about terminal care and so on? It is interesting to note that the claim that terminal care would be disadvantaged is not substantiated on looking at the *actual* QALY figure.

Linda Lamont: I am glad that the possible uses for measures of quality of life are now being considered, even if we cannot yet agree *what* measures to use. I suppose there must be ways of getting at outcomes from the research described today. How much can the work being done on QALYs relate to the standards of care and the users' attitudes to them? Can QALYs help identify the unmet needs? I am still not clear whether we are looking at a defined area of needs when talking about QALYs, or trying to look at the whole spectrum of needs, including those not met in the past.

Another issue I would like to underline is the distinction between looking at what patients and the general public perceive as 'quality of life'. There is also the need to make a distinction between the research being done with people with specific illnesses and how to approach and talk to the public about what they perceive about health. Thirdly, there is the very real problem of getting people to say what their priorities are in situations in which they are not themselves sufferers or carers. In the Oregon experiment, people, most of whom had insurance, were asked to say what should be given to people who did not have insurance.

Participants were asked to indicate how they felt that knowledge in this field could be advanced.

Lesley Fallowfield: Research should explore whether or not clinical and managerial decisions based upon usual clinical information are influenced by the provision of QALY information.

Howard Glennerster: We do such exercises with our students. One week they are presented with QALYs, another week with multiple outcome measures, and a third week with something else—and we have a rather more informed discussion using some of the ideas I have expressed in Chapter 11. With QALYs, at the end of the day, nobody decides anything.

Azim Lakhani: In terms of moving forward, two questions must be considered: first, whether there is a way of measuring the benefit of health care intervention—defining the benefit in a variety of ways. The general consensus seems to be that outcomes to be considered should be more than just changes in clinical signs, symptoms and so on, and should include patients' understanding and values. Secondly, whether, given their understanding and values, this information can then be used for decisions about allocation of resources.

Jack Dowie: An interesting experiment would be to develop a hypothetical budget based on QALY principles for a future year, present it alongside the budget allocation arrived at by the current system, and let the public and other interested parties look at these allocations. If the two methods produce the same results, money spent on QALY work can be saved in the future. If they produce different allocations, I look forward to hearing the discussion.

Ann Bowling: We should start at the beginning and conduct a public survey of attitudes as to what is quality of life, asking people how they define it, and then examine the several dimensions of measures that we have—life satisfaction, social support, depression, disability and so on—to see whether or not these match people's definitions of quality of life in the health-related field. Why not look at half a dozen dimensions of quality of life, score them separately, and look at them in their own right? I know it may be argued that this is cumbersome but, from the social scientist's perspective, this is the only realistic way forward, and it is one which would stop a lot of argument.

Paul Kind: Some strong assertions have been made today about what I might call 'methodological purity'. I have the strong impression that the methodologies and the state of the art within, say, oncology or cardiological medicine is at a stage where there can be some agreement that good reliable measurements of quality of life are available. Since this methodology is in place, there is the potential for new assessments to be run in parallel, and any differences subjected to empirical examination. It would then be possible to argue on the basis of a factual presentation of commonly agreed data and common protocols, and to look again at some of the issues raised at this workshop.

Ian Russell: Martin Buxton pointed out in Chapter 4 that there is the need for comparative evidence from large-scale studies of the results of using different techniques for the same health state descriptions with the same, or directly comparable, respondents. If people working in this field resolved always to use their favourite measure and at least one other, a lot more progress would be made than has happened in the last few years.

Roy Carr-Hill: My suggestion is simpler. I would like to know the impact of using numerical data instead of descriptions of conditions on decision making and on the decisions that are actually taken. There seems to be a presumption that managers, doctors and politicians can decide only on the basis of one number.

Lesley Fallowfield: My sort of research, which is the assessment of the impact of different sorts of treatment upon the quality of life, is very different to the QALY work. It has been confusing today to listen to statements that I thought referred to quality of life measurement as I know it, when in fact they referred to QALYs.

Astrid Fletcher: An area with which I have much difficulty is the integration of quality of life and survival. When cost-effectiveness and cost-utility analyses are carried out in hypertension, I am concerned that the sensitivity of the utilities has a dramatic effect on our decision options. Much of the discussion at this meeting has been geared to the quality of life side of the spectrum and has tended to ignore the other measurements of benefit which, in my example of hypertension, is the prevention of stroke and myocardial infarction.

Summing up

Clive Smee and Anthony Hopkins

Clive Smee: My comments will be confined entirely to decision making in resource allocation. First, different measures of quality of life are needed for different purposes, and recognising this will be a big step towards greater mutual understanding. Secondly, I hope it is recognised that difficult resource allocation decisions have to be made by ministers, managers and clinicians at fairly high levels in the National Health Service who look to us for help. My colleague, Henry Neuberger, has remarked that we are the brokers between clinicians and decision makers. How can we do our brokering more efficiently, or provide those who make the decisions with better information — and where, in particular, do the views of patients come into this?

There is no disagreement that, within the framework of decisions that must be made, measures of quality of life of all kinds are important, and will probably be more so in the future than in the past. What kinds of measures of quality of life may be needed and what is their role relative to other information that should also be put into the decision-making framework? The broader framework of considerations that ministers or health authority members should regard in making decisions has not been discussed.

I think it would be fair to say that the Department of Health has had no formalised and systematic framework for making decisions about resource allocation, no single document which outlines the kinds of considerations that a new administrative trainee should bear in mind. The government has recently produced one in relation to environmental issues, and with such a document it might at least be possible to discuss where measures of quality of life fit into our discussions and the kind of measures of quality of life likely to be most appropriate in different circumstances. Therefore, one item on our agenda is to try to develop a more systematic framework within the Department so that consistent account can be taken of other things that have been discussed here, such as the effects on carers, problems of access, equity and so on. These issues could then be more systematically addressed in advice to senior officials and ministers.

Another important point, which has been mentioned several times, is

143

how to include patients and the public in the decision-making process. I agree with Howard Glennerster that as many decisions as possible should be made by the patients. As others have indicated, this requires informing patients about the range of issues that may be relevant to their future lives and treatment. How this can be done is an important issue for the agenda. I would like to see much more research on the difference made to patients' choices by varying the information they get about the likely outcomes from different interventions.

There should be modesty about the role of measures of quality of life and, where quality-adjusted life years are used, the sensitivity of results should be shown to different assumptions about how quality of life should be weighted relative to length of life. With regard to Astrid Fletcher's point, as in other areas in which decisions are required, ministers' attention should certainly be drawn to the sensitivities.

Where do we go in terms·of the research agenda? Several suggestions (which I will not repeat) have been made, which I hope give departmental officials food for thought. One suggestion that impressed me is that attempts should be made to bring together the measures being developed for clinicians with those being developed or used for higher levels of decision about allocating resources. There should be ways of trying to ensure that we learn from the best of both, and that they are not seen to be in contention and competition. There is tremendous scope for improving the quality of decision making in the health care sector, as well as in other areas of government. At the end of the day, decisions are political, but I do not accept that they cannot be better informed than at present. Moreover, I believe they are likely to be better decisions if better informed.

Anthony Hopkins: I warmly welcome the better efforts that have been made to judge the effectiveness of treatments such as in hypertension (Astrid Fletcher's example) more broadly than just by the reduction in the blood pressure. There must be a continued research endeavour in specific diseases — but the difficulty is that such research does not actually help those concerned in choosing between the different diseases to which resources are allocated. This is Alan Williams' principal point, and one with which I have some sympathy: however perfect our measures for individual diseases, they are of no help in making choices between diseases.

It has been suggested privately that it might have been better to have held two workshops, one to discuss methodological issues and another to discuss ethical issues such as ageism. In practice, I believe it is important that each perspective informs the other. The problem of resource allocation is ever present. There remains a tremendous amount of work to be done.

Appendices

APPENDIX 1
3-Dimensional classification: levels of diagnosis

Disability

D1: No physical disability; perfectly mobile and physically active; able to perform all self-care and role functions.

D2: Slight social disability, eg having slight cold. No limitations with physical ability, self-care or mobility, but some role functions slightly impaired by social disability.

D3: Slight physical disability. Able to get round house and community, but unable to perform heavy physical tasks. Role functions slightly limited by physical disability. Able to perform all self-care activities.

D4: Able to get round house and do lighter physical work. Some difficulty in getting round community due to weakness or other physical limitations. Can perform all self-care activities. Ability to perform role functions limited.

D5: Difficulty in getting round house, can go out only with assistance. Major physical limitations, eg can only do light work. Can perform most self-care activities, but need help getting into and out of bath. Limited ability to perform role functions.

D6: Confined to a chair, therefore can only get out with assistance. Can only do the lightest of tasks, eg switch on the TV. Can feed self, but needs help with all other self-care activities. Very limited ability to perform role functions.

D7: Confined to bed. Needs help with all self-care activities. Minimal ability to perform role functions.

D8: Unconscious.

Discomfort (physical)

P1: No pain.

P2: Slight pain: (a) occasionally, (b) frequently, (c) almost all the time.

147

P3:   Moderate pain: (a) occasionally, (b) frequently, (c) almost all the time.

P4:   Severe pain: (a) occasionally, (b) frequently, (c) almost all the time.

P5:   Agonising pain: (a) occasionally, (b) frequently, (c) almost all the time.

Distress (emotional)

E1:   No distress: very happy and relaxed almost all the time.

E2:   Slight distress: happy and relaxed most of the time, but anxious and depressed some of the time.

E3:   Moderate distress: anxious and depressed most of the time, but happy and relaxed some of the time.

E4:   Severe distress: very anxious and depressed almost all the time.

E5:   Extremely depressed: actively suicidal.

APPENDIX 2
3-Dimensional classification system: composite state valuations (0–1 scale of values)

		E1	E2	E3	E4	E5
P1	D1	1.000	0.970	0.894	0.791	0.643
	D2	0.990	0.960	0.884	0.781	0.632
	D3	0.971	0.940	0.864	0.762	0.614
	D4	0.946	0.917	0.840	0.738	0.590
	D5	0.917	0.887	0.811	0.710	0.561
	D6	0.885	0.855	0.780	0.678	0.530
	D7	0.838	0.804	0.729	0.628	0.481
P2	D1	0.944	0.915	0.838	0.736	0.588
	D2	0.934	0.904	0.828	0.726	0.578
	D3	0.915	0.885	0.810	0.708	0.559
	D4	0.891	0.861	0.785	0.684	0.537
	D5	0.861	0.831	0.756	0.654	0.508
	D6	0.829	0.799	0.724	0.623	0.477
	D7	0.779	0.750	0.675	0.574	0.427
P3	D1	0.867	0.837	0.761	0.660	0.513
	D2	0.857	0.827	0.751	0.650	0.503
	D3	0.837	0.808	0.732	0.631	0.485
	D4	0.814	0.784	0.709	0.608	0.461
	D5	0.785	0.755	0.680	0.579	0.433
	D6	0.753	0.723	0.648	0.548	0.402
	D7	0.702	0.674	0.598	0.498	0.353
P4	D1	0.714	0.685	0.610	0.510	0.365
	D2	0.703	0.675	0.599	0.499	0.354
	D3	0.685	0.656	0.581	0.481	0.337
	D4	0.661	0.632	0.557	0.458	0.313
	D5	0.632	0.604	0.528	0.429	0.285
	D6	0.601	0.572	0.497	0.399	0.254
	D7	0.551	0.522	0.449	0.350	0.207
P5	D1	0.468	0.439	0.365	0.267	0.125
	D2	0.457	0.428	0.355	0.257	0.114
	D3	0.439	0.410	0.337	0.239	0.097
	D4	0.416	0.387	0.314	0.216	0.074
	D5	0.387	0.358	0.285	0.188	0.047
	D6	0.356	0.327	0.255	0.159	0.017
	D7	0.308	0.279	0.207	0.111	−0.030

APPENDIX 3
Hierarchical structure of the IHQL

Due to physical constraints, it is not possible to display the hierarchical structure of the IHQL on a single page. The diagram below shows the top 3 levels (the overall global score, dimensions and attributes) of the hierarchy. The scales and descriptors subsumed by each of the seven attributes are presented on the following three pages.

Alongside each descriptor, the *disutility* values corresponding to different levels of severity are displayed. For example: walk (2 = 0.0052) corresponds to a disutility of 0.0052 for the second level of walk which, although not indicated here, is defined as 'walk: only if assisted' (the definitions of each level of each descriptor are contained in the IHQL questionnaire, copies of which are available from the authors of Chapter 7). For the majority of the descriptors, it is the case that the greater the number assigned to the level (1, 2, 3, etc) then the more severe the problem and the larger the disutility value. 'No problem' always has a disutility value of 0 and is therefore not displayed. By summing the applicable disutility value for every descriptor and subtracting the total from 1, a single value for health-related quality of life is obtained on a 0–1 scale. See Chapter 7 for more details.

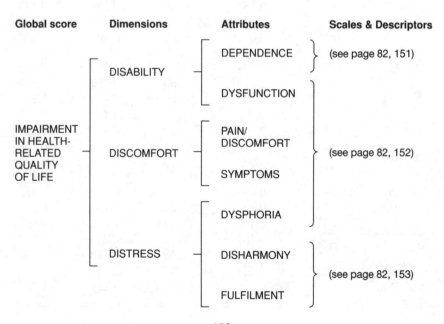

Attribute	Scale	Descriptor	Values
DEPENDENCE	Self-care	wash	(2=0.0062) (1=0.0038)
		dress	(2=0.0055) (1=0.0032)
		feed	(2=0.0065) (1=0.0043)
	Mobility	walk	(3=0.0085) (2=0.0052) (1=0.0031)
		travel	(3=0.0079) (2=0.0046) (1=0.0017)
	Physical disability	paralysis	(2=0.0043) (1=0.0020)
		weakness	(2=0.0031) (1=0.0011)
		stiffness	(2=0.0027) (1=0.0010)
		amputation	(2=0.0042) (1=0.0021)
		involuntary movements	(2=0.0035) (1=0.0015)
		tremor	(2=0.0030) (1=0.0012)
	Treatment away from home	general hospital	(1=0.0091)
		psychiatric unit	(2=0.0124)
		mental hospital	(3=0.0142)
		intensive care unit	(4=0.0204)
		hospice	(5=0.0110)
		hostel	(6=0.0068)
	Cognitive Function	thought disorder	(2=0.0031) (1=0.0017)
		memory loss	(4=0.0032) (3=0.0028) (2=0.0021) (1=0.0011)
		loss of concentration	(4=0.0028) (3=0.0024)
		confusion	(4=0.0032) (2=0.0016) (1=0.0008)
		disorientation in time	(2=0.0028) (1=0.0012)
		disorientation in place	(2=0.0028) (1=0.0014)
		disorientation in person	(2=0.0031) (1=0.0018)
	Consciousness	unconscious	(2=0.0241) (1=0.0130)
		other impairment	(2=0.0188) (1=0.0125)
	Vegetative Function	incontinent of bowel	(2=0.0054) (1=0.0037)
		incontinent of bladder	(2=0.0047) (1=0.0029)
		machine inside body	(2=0.0031) (1=0.0016)
		machine outside body	(2=0.0046) (1=0.0023)
		reliant on a transplant	(1=0.0031)
		prescribed drugs	(1=0.0028)
		addictive drugs	(1=0.0061)
		mind affecting drugs	(1=0.0067)
	Sensory Deficits	sight	(3=0.0066) (2=0.0035) (1=0.0015)
		hearing	(3=0.0061) (2=0.0033) (1=0.0015)
		touch	(3=0.0031) (2=0.0018) (1=0.0008)
		smell	(3=0.0031) (2=0.0014) (1=0.0005)
		taste	(3=0.0034) (2=0.0016) (1=0.0007)

ATTRIBUTES   SCALES & DESCRIPTORS

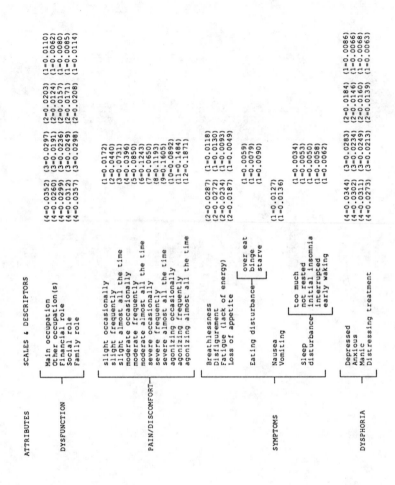

ATTRIBUTES　　SCALES & DESCRIPTORS

DYSFUNCTION
Main occupation　　　(4=0.0352) (3=0.0297) (2=0.0203) (1=0.0110)
Other occupation(s)　(4=0.0260) (3=0.0191) (2=0.0124) (1=0.0062)
Financial role　　　 (4=0.0299) (3=0.0236) (2=0.0157) (1=0.0080)
Social role　　　　　(4=0.0312) (3=0.0249) (2=0.0171) (1=0.0085)
Family role　　　　　(4=0.0357) (3=0.0298) (2=0.0208) (1=0.0114)

PAIN/DISCOMFORT
slight occasionally　　　　　　 (1=0.0172)
slight frequently　　　　　　　 (2=0.0440)
slight almost all the time　　　(3=0.0731)
moderate occasionally　　　　　 (4=0.0396)
moderate frequently　　　　　　 (5=0.0850)
moderate almost all the time　 (6=0.1243)
severe occasionally　　　　　　 (7=0.0650)
severe frequently　　　　　　　 (8=0.1193)
severe almost all the time　　　(9=0.1605)
agonizing occasionally　　　　 (10=0.0892)
agonizing frequently　　　　　 (11=0.1484)
agonizing almost all the time (12=0.1871)

SYMPTOMS
Breathlessness　　　　　　 (2=0.0287) (1=0.0118)
Disfigurement　　　　　　　(2=0.0272) (1=0.0130)
Fatigue (lack of energy)　(2=0.0234) (1=0.0093)
Loss of appetite　　　　　 (2=0.0187) (1=0.0049)

Eating disturbance ⎰ over eat　 (1=0.0059)
　　　　　　　　　　 ⎱ binge　　　(1=0.0079)
　　　　　　　　　　 ⎱ starve　　 (1=0.0090)

Nausea　　(1=0.0127)
Vomiting　(1=0.0136)

Sleep disturbance ⎰ too much　　　　 (1=0.0034)
　　　　　　　　　　 ⎱ not rested　　　 (1=0.0053)
　　　　　　　　　　 ⎱ initial insomnia (1=0.0050)
　　　　　　　　　　 ⎱ interrupted　　　(1=0.0058)
　　　　　　　　　　 ⎱ early waking　　 (1=0.0062)

DYSPHORIA
Depressed　　　　　　 (4=0.0344) (3=0.0283) (2=0.0184) (1=0.0086)
Anxious　　　　　　　 (4=0.0302) (3=0.0234) (2=0.0146) (1=0.0066)
Manic　　　　　　　　 (4=0.0311) (3=0.0249) (2=0.0160) (1=0.0068)
Distressing treatment (4=0.0273) (3=0.0213) (2=0.0139) (1=0.0063)

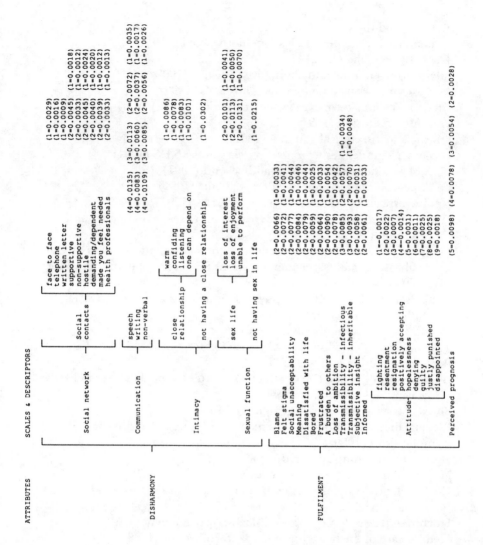

Reports of the Royal College of Physicians

Smoking and the young (1992)
Standardised assessment scales for elderly people (1992)
The CARE scheme (1992)
Allergy: conventional and alternative concepts (1992)
A charter for disabled people using hospitals (1992)
High quality long-term care for elderly people (1992)
Preventive medicine (1991)
Ethical issues in clinical genetics (1991)
Purchaser's guidelines to genetic services in the NHS (1991)
Clinical genetic services in 1990 and beyond (1991)
Cardiological intervention in elderly patients (1991)
Medical aspects of exercise: benefits and risks (1991)
Fraud and misconduct in medical research: causes, investigation and
    prevention (1991)
Compensation for adverse consequences of medical intervention (1990)
Cystic fibrosis in adults: recommendations for care of patients in the UK
    (1990)
Health services for adults with physical disabilities: a survey of district
    health authorities 1988/89 (1990)
Training in infectious diseases (1990)
Teaching genetics to medical students (1990)
Research involving patients (1990)
Guidelines on the practice of ethics committees in medical research
    involving human subjects (1990)
Stroke: towards better management (1989)
Prenatal diagnosis and genetic screening: community and service
    implications (1989)
Hay fever (including abridged version) (1989)
Medical audit: a first report – what, why and how? (1989)
Care of elderly people with mental illness: specialist services and medical
    training (1989)
Fractured neck of femur: prevention and management (1989)
Medical care of the newborn in England and Wales (1988)
Resuscitation from cardiopulmonary arrest: training and organisation
    (1987)
Links between exposure to ultraviolet radiation and skin cancer (1987)
The sun on your skin (*an abridged version of the above Report*) (1987)
Physical disability in 1986 and beyond (1986)
The young disabled adult (1986)
Research on healthy volunteers (1986)
The relationship between physicians and the pharmaceutical industry
    (1986)
A great and growing evil: the medical consequences of alcohol abuse
    (1986)
Health or Smoking (1983)

All available from the College